P9-BID-202

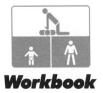

American Red Cross CPR: Infant and Child

Workbook

© 1988 by The American National Red Cross
All Rights Reserved

This workbook is an integral part of the
American Red Cross CPR: Infant and Child course.
By itself, it does not constitute adequate training for first aid.
Please contact your local Red Cross chapter
for more information on this course.

ISBN: 0-86536-135-5

Acknowledgments

This course is based on the Standards and Guidelines established by the 1985 National Conference on Cardiopulmonary Resuscitation and Emergency Cardiac Care.

The course and this workbook are products of the 1987–1988 CPR/First Aid Project at American Red Cross national headquarters. The team that developed this course included M. Elizabeth Buoy, M.P.H.; Valerie W. Drake, M.A.; Lawrence Newell, Ed.D.; and Suzanne M. Randolph, Ph.D. Additional assistance was provided by Program Development staff, including Bruce Spitz, director; Frank Carroll; Mary F. Cotton, Ph.D.; Jessica Bernstein, M.P.H.; Karen Peterson, Ph.D.; Victoria Scott, M.P.A.; Pamela B. Mangu, M.A.; and Susan Walter. The following national sector staff also provided assistance: Joan Handler; Alfred J. Katz, M.D.; Carole Kauffman, R.N., M.P.H.; John M. Malatak, M.S.; and Donald Miller, J.D.

Technical advice and review were provided by the following:

Susan Aronson, M.D., F.A.A.P., Practicing Pediatrician; Clinical Professor of Pediatrics at Hahnemann University, Philadelphia, Pa.

Allan Braslow, Ph.D., Faculty, 1985 National Conference on Cardiopulmonary Resuscitation and Emergency Cardiac Care; Braslow & Associates.

Sandra E. Clarke, S.C.C., Executive Director, Advanced Coronary Treatment (ACT) Foundation of Canada, Ottawa, Ont.

Ellen Galinsky, Project Director, Work and Family Life Studies, Division of Research, Demonstration and Policy, Bank Street College of Education, New York, N.Y.

Pearl L. Rosser, M.D., F.A.A.P., Practicing Pediatrician; former Director, Howard University Child Development Center, Washington, D.C.

William J. Schneiderman, Assistant Director, Medic IV Emergency Medical Services Project, Massachusetts Hospital Association, Burlington, Mass.

James Seidel, M.D., Ph.D., Associate Professor and Chief of Ambulatory Pediatrics, University of California at Los Angeles Medical Center, Torrance, Calif.

Mark D. Widome, M.D., Chairman, Committee on Accident and Poison Prevention, American Academy of Pediatrics, Hershey, Pa.

Material in this manuscript was reviewed by the National Academy of Sciences–National Research Council Committee to Advise the American National Red Cross.

Field representatives who provided advice and guidance through the 1987–1988 Red Cross CPR Advisory Committee included the following:

W. Larry Bair, Central Iowa Chapter, Des Moines, Iowa.

D. Earl Harbert, Field Service Manager, Wichita, Kan.

Jerry Hummel, Southeastern Michigan Chapter, Detroit, Mich.

Lonnie Kirby, Western Operations Headquarters, Burlingame, Calif.

Wanda Leffler, Indianapolis Area Chapter, Indianapolis, Ind.

Mary M. "Posie" Mansfield, Danvers, Mass.; Chair, Basic Life Support Subcommittee of the CPR Advisory Committee.

C. Ray McLain, R.N., M.S.N., Assistant Professor, University of Alabama, Birmingham, Ala.; Chairman, Infant/Child CPR Subcommittee of the CPR Advisory Committee.

Marshall Meyer, Oregon Trail Chapter, Portland, Oreg.

Gary J. Taylor, Greater Kansas City Chapter, Kansas City, Mo.

Richard Tulis, American Red Cross of Massachusetts Bay, Boston, Mass.

John Wagner, Albany Area Chapter, Albany, N.Y.

Red Cross chapters that participated in pilot and field tests included the following:

Alachua County Chapter, Gainesville, Fla.

American Red Cross of Massachusetts Bay, Boston, Mass.

American Red Cross San Francisco Bay Area, San Francisco, Calif.

Birmingham Area Chapter, Birmingham, Ala.

Dallas Area Chapter, Dallas, Tex.

Louisiana Capital Area Chapter, Baton Rouge, La.

Midway-Kansas Chapter, Wichita, Kan.

Pikes Peak Chapter, Colorado Springs, Colo.

Southeastern Massachusetts Chapter, Brockton, Mass.

Contents

Why the American Red Cross Teaches This Course

This course will teach you lifesaving skills to help infants and children. You need these skills when a breathing or cardiac emergency happens. A breathing emergency is a situation in which it is difficult or impossible for a person to breathe, such as choking or near-drowning. A cardiac emergency is a situation in which a person's heart stops beating or is not beating properly.

This course will help you learn the early signals of a breathing emergency. When a breathing emergency occurs, it is up to you to recognize that emergency medical help is needed, to begin first aid, and to phone the emergency medical services (EMS) system for help. By giving first aid in a breathing emergency, you may prevent a cardiac emergency that might have led to death. In this course, you will learn how to deal with an emergency, and how to give first aid until advanced emergency medical care arrives.

This course will teach you—

1. How to give first aid when an infant or child stops breathing.
2. How to give first aid for choking to an infant and to a child.
3. How to give CPR to an infant or child whose heart has stopped.
4. How to use the emergency medical services (EMS) system.
5. How to reduce the risk of injury to infants and children.

First, you will learn skills to help children. These skills should be used to help a child, a person age one through eight years old. Then you will learn skills to help an infant, a person younger than one year old.

The following parts of the course have been designed to help you learn these skills.

Video/Film
During this course you will see short videos or films. These show you the skills you will practice. Watching the video or film carefully will help you do well when you practice.

Practice Sessions
After you watch a video or film, you will learn each skill by practicing it. You will work with a partner. You will practice the skills on manikins.

Workbook
You will not be required to read the entire workbook during class. However, you will use the workbook for practice sessions. The chapters describe the skills you will learn. The illustrations show you how to do each skill. The workbook also has the following helpful features:

> **Objectives**
> Each chapter in the workbook begins with a list of objectives. The objectives tell you what you should be able to do after reading the chapter.

Review Questions

There are review questions in each chapter. You can use these questions to check how well you are learning. Answering these questions will help you prepare for the final written test. The correct answers are on the page after each set of questions. Turn the page to check your answers. Change any wrong answers.

Review Sections

Some chapters have a review section at the end. You will use the review sections to check yourself after you have practiced the skills. The answers to the questions in the review section are on the page following the questions.

Skill Sheets

Some chapters have skill sheets. Skill sheets tell how to do first aid skills. The skill sheets also have pictures to show you how to do each skill. You will use the skill sheets when you practice the skills.

Glossary

The glossary explains the meaning of words used in the book. The glossary is found on pages 195 and 196.

Appendixes

There are two appendixes. One gives information about the emergency medical services (EMS) system. The other is a Home Safety Checklist. You can use this to check your home for dangers to infants and children.

Tests

There are two kinds of tests in this course: skill tests and a written test. You will take a skill test after you have practiced each skill. You will take a written test at the end of the course. It is a multiple-choice test about things you have learned in the course.

Some Health Precautions and Guidelines to Follow During This Course

Infection and Disease

Since the beginning of citizen training in CPR (**cardiopulmonary resuscitation**), the American Red Cross and the American Heart Association have trained more than 50 million people in the lifesaving skills contained in this text. According to the Centers for Disease Control (CDC), there has never been a reported case of any infectious disease transmitted through the use of CPR manikins. This is partially due to the standards followed in the manikin decontamination procedure during and after class.

Red Cross chapters have been given guidelines, provided by the Centers for Disease Control, for decontaminating manikins used in CPR training. If these guidelines are followed, there is no known risk of disease transmission. Additionally, we ask the course participants to observe the following guidelines:

Do not use the training manikin—

- If you have any cuts or sores on your hands, head, face, lips, or mouth (for example, cold sores).
- If you are known to be seropositive for hepatitis B surface antigen (HBsAG).
- If you have any respiratory infections, such as a cold or a sore throat.
- If you are infected by the AIDS (acquired immune deficiency syndrome) virus or have AIDs.
- If you have recently been exposed to or are showing symptoms of any infectious disease.

To protect yourself and other students from infection, you should do the following:

- Wash your hands thoroughly before working with the manikin.
- Do not eat, drink, or use tobacco products immediately before or during manikin use.
- Before you use the manikin, dry the manikin's face with a clean gauze pad. Next, vigorously wipe the manikin's face and the inside of its mouth with a clean gauze pad soaked with a solution of household bleach and water (sodium hypochlorite and water) or rubbing alcohol. Place this wet pad over the manikin's mouth and nose and wait for at least 30 seconds before you wipe the face dry with a clean gauze pad.
- When practicing what to do for a blocked airway, simulate (pretend to do) the finger sweep.

Physical Stress and Injury

CPR requires strenuous activity. If you have a medical condition or disability that will prevent you from taking part in the practice sessions, please let your instructor know.

Damage to Manikins

In order to protect the manikins from damage, you should do the following before you begin to practice:

- Remove pens and pencils from your pockets.
- Remove all jewelry.
- Remove lipstick and excess makeup.
- Remove chewing gum and candy from your mouth.

How Much Do You Know About Childhood Emergencies?

Here are some questions about childhood emergencies. The questions will help you think about what can cause an emergency. They will help you think about what you can do to help a child who is sick or hurt. They will help you think about how to prevent such emergencies.

Choose the best answer for each question. Then read the correct answers. Don't expect to answer every question correctly.

1. What is the leading cause of death in children in the U.S.?
    ☐ Injury from accidents
    ☐ Cancer

2. What is the safest way for a toddler to ride in a car?
    ☐ Sitting on someone's lap
    ☐ Buckled into an adult seat belt
    ☐ Buckled into a car safety seat

3. An infant is choking on a piece of food. She cannot cough, cry, or breathe. What should you do?
    ☐ Give her a drink of water.
    ☐ Give her back blows and chest thrusts.

4. While shopping, you hear a yell for help. You see a mother with a child in a cart. The child is coughing weakly. The mother says, "He was eating some candy." What should you do?
    ☐ Run to get help.
    ☐ Give the child abdominal thrusts.
    ☐ Hold him upside down by the ankles and shake him.

5. What does CPR do for a person whose heart has stopped beating?
    ☐ CPR restarts the heart.
    ☐ CPR supplies oxygen to every part of the body.

6. You find an infant lying on his back in his crib. He is not moving. You gently shake his shoulder, but he doesn't move or make a noise. You shout for help. What should you do next?
    ☐ Check to see if he is breathing and has a pulse.
    ☐ Call for an ambulance.

Answers

1. **Injury from accidents** is the leading cause of death in children in the United States. A child is much more likely to die from an injury than from cancer or another disease.

2. The safest way for a toddler to ride in a car is **buckled into a car safety seat.** A car safety seat will hold a child in place if there is a car accident. You can prevent a toddler from being injured or killed by buckling the child into a car safety seat on each and every ride.

3. If an infant chokes on a piece of food and cannot cough, cry, or breathe, **give back blows and chest thrusts.** Chapter 7 describes the first aid for an infant who is choking.

4. You should **give abdominal thrusts** to a conscious child who is choking. Chapter 4 describes the first aid for a child who is choking.

5. **CPR supplies oxygen to every part of the body** when the heart has stopped beating. CPR does not restart the heart. CPR works because you breathe air into the person's lungs to get air into the blood. Then, when you press on the chest, you move oxygen-carrying blood through the body. Chapter 5 describes how to give CPR to a child. Chapter 8 shows you how to give CPR to an infant.

6. **Check to see if the infant is breathing and has a pulse.** You should do this before you phone for an ambulance. You should tell the emergency medical services dispatcher whether the infant is breathing and has a pulse. In this course, you will learn what to do in an emergency. Chapter 2 describes the emergency action principles. You should follow these steps to deal with an emergency.

What This Course Will Teach You

Sixteen-year-old Trisha was babysitting for her neighbors, the Johnsons. The two Johnson boys, Shawn and Mike, were watching TV in the living room. Trisha went into the kitchen to answer the telephone.

Suddenly seven-year-old Shawn ran into the kitchen. "Trisha, come quick! Something's wrong with Mike!" he shouted. Trisha raced into the living room. Two-year-old Mike was turning blue. He could not talk and was grasping at his throat. Trisha caught him as he became unconscious and fell to the floor. Mike had stopped breathing.

Would You Know What to Do?

If you were in Trisha's place, would you know what to do? Would you be able to tell what was wrong with Mike? Would you be able to give the correct first aid? In this course, you will learn what to do in a life-threatening emergency. You will learn what to do if a child or infant stops breathing. You will learn first aid for a child or infant who is choking. You will learn how to give CPR to a child or infant whose heart has stopped beating.

Injury Is the Number One Killer

Injury from accidents is the leading cause of death in children ages one through 14. A child is much more likely to die from an injury than from a disease. For infants less than one year old, injury from accidents is the fourth leading cause of death.

Each year thousands of children in the United States are killed in accidents. Millions of children under 15 years of age need medical care for accidental injuries.

Reducing Childhood Deaths and Injuries

Many deaths and injuries to children and infants could be prevented. In this course you will learn how to protect children by removing dangers, giving supervision, and teaching safety rules and safety habits.

You will also learn what to do when an infant or child is injured. This course is designed to help you recognize when an infant or child needs first aid. For example, you will learn to recognize when a child may be about to stop breathing. By recognizing a breathing emergency and giving first aid, you may be able to save the child's life.

In an emergency, a child's life may depend on whether you can give first aid and call for emergency medical services. When a child's heart stops beating, the child needs CPR right away. Advanced emergency medical care should be started within 10 minutes.

Your Role as a Rescuer

Rescuers—citizens like you—play a vital role in giving first aid. It is up to you to recognize a life-threatening emergency. You must begin first aid and alert your community's emergency medical services (EMS) system. You must provide the important information the EMS dispatcher needs to send the right help quickly.

As a trained rescuer, you will be part of the EMS system. The other parts of the EMS system include trained emergency medical personnel, special equipment, and communications systems. EMS systems vary from one community to another. Find out about the EMS system in your community before an emergency happens. Learn the telephone number for the EMS system. Many communities use 911. Learn about the type of care your EMS system can give. To learn more about how an EMS system works, read the appendix on pages 186 through 190 of this workbook.

In an emergency, minutes count. Knowing about the EMS system and how to give first aid can help you make the right decisions. You can quickly phone the EMS system, give important information, and provide first aid until EMS personnel arrive.

A Happy Ending

Now let's go back to the story at the beginning of this section. Mike was lucky. Trisha was a trained rescuer. In her high school health class, she had learned first aid skills. Trisha recognized that Mike was choking. She had Shawn call the EMS system. She gave Mike abdominal thrusts. Then she looked in his mouth and saw something. She was able to remove the object with her finger. The boy began to breathe on his own. Mike had choked on a piece of food.

A few minutes later an ambulance arrived, and the trained personnel took over. The boy would live, thanks to Trisha who knew what to do in an emergency.

1 *What You Can Do to Prevent Childhood Injuries*

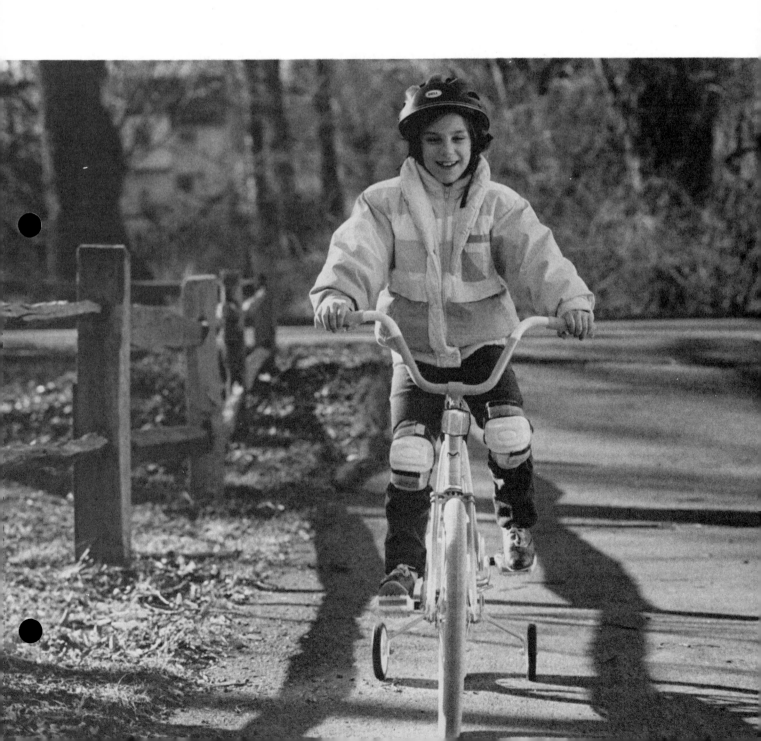

This chapter will help you think about safety. You will learn what you can do to prevent injuries to children.

Objectives

By the time you finish reading this chapter, you should be able to do the following:
1. *Name the major causes of injuries to infants and children.*
2. *List the three basic parts of an injury-prevention plan.*
3. *Describe injury-prevention plans for children of different ages and stages of development.*

Becoming Safety Conscious

Parents do many things to keep their children healthy, like giving them good foods and taking them for checkups. Parents try to keep their children from getting sick. Children are given shots to prevent measles, mumps, and other diseases. But in the United States, sickness is not the greatest threat to the health of young children. The number one killer of young children is injury. Each year about 8,000 children die from injuries. Thousands more children are treated in hospitals for injuries. Many of these deaths and injuries could be prevented.

There are three ways that you can help prevent injuries to children. One is to keep children away from things that might harm them. For example, don't let a child play with a carving knife. The second way is to stay near children so that you can act in case of danger. For example, if you are bathing a toddler, stay beside the tub so you can catch the child in case of a fall. The third way is to follow safety rules yourself and teach them to children. For example, cross streets with a green light or walk signal. Teach children to wait for the green light and look for cars before crossing.

Later in this chapter, you will learn how to develop a plan. Use this plan to prevent injuries to your own children, if you are a parent, or to other children who are in your care.

But first, think about some general safety rules. These rules will help you protect children of all ages. Later, you will read about safety rules for children in three age groups.

General Safety Rules

Here are some safety rules you should follow to protect children:

1. Think ahead, expect danger.
2. Always expect children to be curious.
3. "Buckle up" children in motor vehicles.
4. Always supervise children in or near water.
5. Check your home for fire and burn dangers.
6. Be prepared for an emergency.

Let's take a closer look at these rules to see what they mean.

1. Think ahead, expect danger

   Think about how injuries might happen. Think about how a child might be injured. Then, do whatever you can to reduce the risk of injury. For example, a child who is riding a bicycle might fall off or be hit by a car. To protect this child, you could buy a helmet for him or her to wear when riding a bicycle. Make sure the bicycle is the correct size for the rider and has no broken parts *(Fig. 1)*.

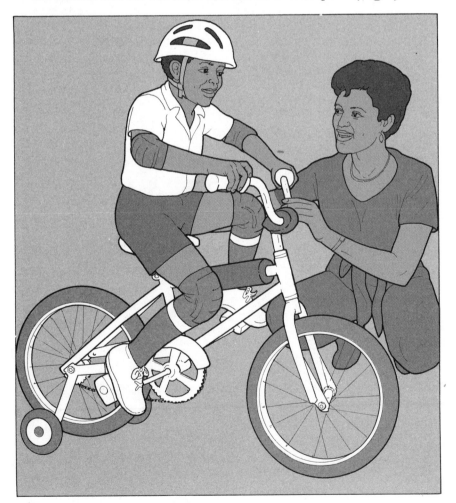

Figure 1
Think Ahead to Prevent Injuries

11

2. Always expect children to be curious

Children like to explore. They like to touch, taste, poke, pull, reach, and climb. As they grow, they are able to do more. This can get them into danger. To protect children from injury, you must remember their love of exploring. You must also remember that a child's abilities change quickly.

3. "Buckle up" children in motor vehicles

Infants and young children should always be buckled into approved car safety seats *(Fig. 2)*. They should never ride in a passenger's arms. Buy or rent a car seat. Install and use the seat correctly, following the manufacturer's directions. As children grow, they will use a car safety seat, then a booster seat, and finally adult safety belts. The important thing is that children should always be in the correct car seat and/or safety belt for their age and size.

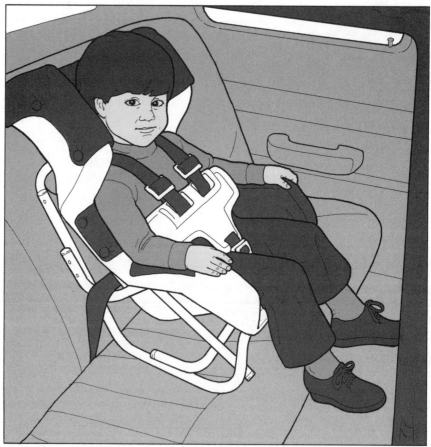

Figure 2
"Buckle up" Children in Motor Vehicles

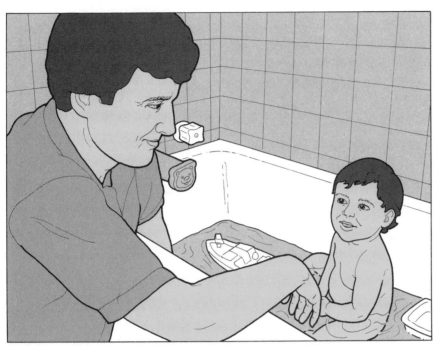

Figure 3
**Always Supervise Children in
Water**

4. **Always supervise children in or near water**
   Young children can drown in as little as two inches of water.
   Never leave young children alone in or near a bathtub, wading or
   swimming pool, pond, or any other body of water *(Fig. 3)*.

5. **Check your home for fire and burn dangers**
   Take steps to prevent fires. Make sure that the electrical wiring in
   your home meets safety codes. Install smoke detectors to warn
   you if a fire starts. Check smoke detectors often to make sure they
   work. To lower the risk of tap water burns, turn your hot water
   heater to 120°F.

6. **Be prepared for an emergency**
   Place fire extinguishers where a fire is most likely to happen, such
   as the kitchen. Make a plan for leaving your home in case of fire.
   Have fire drills. Take a Red Cross first aid course.

Prepare for poisoning emergencies by buying syrup of ipecac at a drugstore. Syrup of ipecac is used in some cases of poisoning to make a child vomit. If you suspect that a child has been poisoned, telephone your area poison control center.

Post a list of emergency numbers by each telephone in the home. You can use the form, "Instructions for Emergency Calls," found on the last page of this book. This list should include the following numbers:

- Emergency medical services (EMS) system
- Fire department
- Police department
- Poison control center
- Parents' work
- Physician
- Close neighbor

Developing an Injury-Prevention Plan

To help prevent injury, you must make a child's world safer. The six safety rules you just read are general guidelines. The rest of this chapter will tell you how to prevent injuries to children in three age groups:

- Infants—from birth to age one
- Toddlers and preschoolers—ages one to five
- Young school-age children—ages five to nine

Each age group is different. As children grow, they quickly learn new skills. What they can do and what they want to do quickly changes. These changing abilities and interests can lead children into danger. Adults must protect children by reducing the risk of injury.

An injury-prevention plan can help prevent injuries. A good plan must match the age of the child you want to protect. This chapter includes three injury-prevention plans: one for infants, one for toddlers and preschoolers, and one for young school-age children. The first plan tells you how to make an infant's world safer. The second plan tells you how to protect toddlers and preschoolers. The third plan shows how to keep young school-age children from being injured.

Each injury-prevention plan is divided into three parts as follows:

1. **Remove dangers**

    Where there is a danger, there is a chance that someone will be injured. For example, a bottle of poisonous furniture polish stored under a kitchen sink is a danger to a toddler. It is possible that the child will drink the polish and be poisoned. The danger can easily be removed by storing the polish where the child cannot reach it.

2. **Give supervision**

   Supervision means watching over a child and knowing what the child is doing all the time. This means that you or someone else is always with the child or nearby. Children are often injured when they are left alone for just a few minutes. Supervision is an important part of keeping a child safe. The amount of supervision needed changes as a child grows and develops.

3. **Teach safety**

   You can teach safety in two ways. First, you can set an example of safe behavior by acting safely yourself. Second, you can encourage children to act safely, showing them what they **should do.** For example, make sure children always buckle their seat belts. You should also teach them what they **should not do.** For example, teach children that they should not touch a hot stove. But remember, it takes time to learn safe behavior and to make it a habit.

Preventing Injuries to Infants

About Infants

When infants are born, their parents and other adults must do everything for them. But from birth, infants learn how to control their body. Newborn infants wiggle and wave their arms and legs. Soon they learn to lift their head, roll over, and grab things. Later they learn how to sit, crawl, and stand. With each new skill, they can learn more by moving and touching, hearing, seeing, and tasting.

Infants learn about their world by putting objects in their mouth. They grasp and pull with their hands. This can lead them into danger. The infant who can wiggle can roll off a bed and break a leg. The infant who can pick up a button or bead can put it in his or her mouth and choke. The infant who can pull things from a table can be burned by a cup of hot coffee. Infants face new dangers as they learn to roll, creep and crawl, stand, climb, and walk. But they cannot recognize danger, and it is up to adults to protect them.

Some of the steps that parents and other caregivers can take to prevent injuries to infants are shown in the chart, "What You Can Do to Prevent Injuries to Infants." As you read this chart, keep in mind that for infants motor vehicle accidents are a leading cause of death from injuries. Other common injuries are choking, suffocation, burns and injuries from house fires, near-drowning, falls, and poisoning.

The chart shows you some of the ways you can reduce the risk of injury and death in infants. Use the chart to make your own injury-prevention plan.

What You Can Do to Prevent Injuries to Infants

Injury Risks	Prevention Steps
Car-related	**1. Remove Dangers** Buckle infants into car safety seat on each and every ride. Use only an approved car safety seat. Install the safety seat correctly. The seat should face the rear of the car until the infant weighs about 20 pounds.
Choking	Don't leave small objects (buttons, coins, beads, small pieces of older children's toys, etc.) within an infant's reach. Check infants' toys to make sure they are too large to be swallowed and have no small, detachable parts like buttons. Give infants soft food that does not require chewing. Cut food for older infants into small pieces, especially food like hot dogs. Do not give infants nuts, raw vegetables, popcorn, etc.
Suffocation/ Strangulation	Keep plastic bags and filmy plastic away from infants. Use a crib with slats 2⅜ inches apart or less and a snug-fitting mattress. Keep furniture such as cribs, play pens, and high chairs away from drapery cords and electric appliance cords. Never hang rattles, pacifiers, or other objects around an infant's neck. If an infant can sit up, don't hang toys across the crib.
Burns and House Fires	Check your home for fire hazards. (Ask your local fire department for help with this.) Set the thermostat on water heater to 120°F. Install smoke detectors and keep them in working order by testing them and replacing batteries when needed. Check the bathwater temperature to make sure it is not too hot. Do not cook while holding an infant. Keep hot foods and liquids and lit cigarettes out of an infant's reach. Keep handles on pots and pans turned to the back of the stove when you cook. Put barriers around fireplaces, radiators, hot pipes, wood-burning stoves, and other hot surfaces to separate infants from them. Place high chairs away from stoves. Make sure the electric cords of irons, coffee makers, and other hot appliances are not hanging from counters. Put safety covers or tape on electric outlets. Buy flame-resistant clothing, especially sleepwear.
Falls	Stay with an infant who is on a bed or changing table. Put barriers at the top and bottom of stairs before an infant begins to creep and crawl.

Injury Risks	Prevention Steps
Falls (*continued*)	Hold the handrail when you carry an infant down the stairs. Use skidproof mats or stickers in the bathtub. Keep stairways clear of objects that could cause you to fall while holding an infant. Choose a high chair that is stable and wide-based and that has a seat belt. Be sure all low windows are locked and well screened.
Poisoning	Use nontoxic finishes and lead-free paint when painting and refinishing toys and infants' furniture. Store all prescription and nonprescription medicines in locked cupboards. Keep all medicines in original containers. Store alcohol in locked cabinets. Keep house plants out of reach. See that all handbags, including those of visiting friends and relatives, are out of reach. Buy a bottle of syrup of ipecac to be used as directed in case of poisoning. Keep cleaning supplies in original containers and store them out of reach. Keep cosmetics such as nail polish and hair spray out of reach. Store basement and garage supplies such as moth balls, paints, and fertilizers out of reach.
Drowning (both indoors and outdoors) **Falls** **Choking**	**2. Give Supervision** Stay with infants while they are in or near water, whether in the tub or in a wading or swimming pool. Do not leave an infant in an infant seat alone when the infant seat is on a table or counter. Stay with an infant on a bed or changing table. Never leave a bottle propped up for an infant to drink unsupervised.
General	**3. Teach Safety** Use your tone of voice and simple phrases such as "No, don't touch" and "Not for baby" as a start to safety education for your infant. Behave safely yourself.

Preventing Injuries to Toddlers and Preschoolers

About Toddlers and Preschoolers

Like infants, toddlers and preschoolers are always exploring and trying new things. But toddlers and preschoolers are very different from infants. They can walk and do more with their body than infants can. They can use words to ask for things and talk to other people.

Toddlers and preschoolers are also very different from adults. Toddlers do not realize that what happens to them in one situation might happen to them in a similar situation. A toddler who falls off a fence once will probably continue to climb and fall. The toddler is not able to think, "If I climb that fence, I might fall and hurt myself." This is why supervision is important. Toddlers and preschoolers need simple, clear instructions such as, "Don't climb the fence." Remind them often about what they should and should not do.

Some of the steps that parents and other caregivers can take to keep toddlers and preschoolers safe are shown in the chart, "What You Can Do to Prevent Injuries to Toddlers and Preschoolers." As you read this chart, keep in mind that motor vehicle accidents are the leading cause of injury and death to children in this age group. Other common injuries are near-drowning, burns and injuries from house fires, choking, falls, and poisoning. The chart shows you some of the ways you can reduce the risk of injuries to toddlers and preschoolers. Use the chart to make your own injury-prevention plan.

What You Can Do to Prevent Injuries to Toddlers and Preschoolers

Injury Risks	Prevention Steps
Car-related	**1. Remove Dangers** Buckle toddlers and preschoolers into approved car safety seats on each and every ride. Use only an approved car safety seat. Install the safety seat correctly. Make sure toddlers and preschoolers play in areas separated from traffic.
Burns and House Fires	Check your home for fire dangers. (Ask your fire department for help with this.) Set thermostat on hot water heater to 120°F. Install smoke detectors and keep them in working order by testing them and replacing batteries when needed. Check bathwater temperature to make sure it is not too hot. Keep electric cords out of toddlers' and preschoolers' reach. Keep toddlers and preschoolers away from the stove, iron, and other dangerous appliances. Put safety covers on electric outlets, and move furniture so that outlets are not easily seen or touched. Keep hot foods and liquids and lit cigarettes out of reach. Keep matches, lighters, and cigarettes out of small children's sight and reach. Put barriers around fireplaces, radiators, hot pipes, and other hot surfaces to separate children from them. Buy flame-resistant clothing, especially sleepwear.
Choking	Choose toys that are too large to be swallowed and that have no small, detachable parts. Do not give toddlers and preschoolers nuts, popcorn, raw vegetables, and other foods that could cause choking. Cut foods such as hot dogs into small pieces. Seat toddlers and preschoolers in a high chair or at a table for meals and snacks.
Falls	Check to be sure playground equipment is in good condition. Sand or cedar chips under play equipment make it safer. Put barriers at the top and bottom of stairs until toddlers show that they are steady on their feet and can use handrails properly. Make household rugs skidproof. Use skidproof mats or stickers in the bathtub. Don't give children toys with sharp edges or points.

What You Can Do to Prevent Injuries to Toddlers and Preschoolers

Injury Risks	Prevention Steps
Falls (*continued*)	Cushion sharp edges of furniture with cotton and masking tape or commercial corner guards. Keep doors to porches, attics, laundry rooms, and basements locked. Put window guards in rooms above the first floor. Be sure all low windows are locked and well screened. Lock the sides of a crib at the highest level and put the mattress at the lowest level to prevent a child from climbing out.
Poisoning	Keep all medicines in original containers. Store all medicines in a locked cabinet, your shoulder height or higher. Keep house plants out of reach. Buy a bottle of syrup of ipecac to be used as directed in case of poisoning. Store alcohol in locked cabinets. Keep cosmetics, such as nail polish and hair spray, out of reach. Keep cleaning supplies in original containers and store them out of reach and out of sight. Store basement and garage supplies such as moth balls, paints, and fertilizers out of reach. See that all handbags are out of reach. Always use nontoxic finishes and lead-free paint on toys and furniture.
Drowning	If you have a home swimming pool, fence it completely around to prevent access from the house by your child.
Drowning (both indoors and outdoors)	**2. Give Supervision** Stay with toddlers and preschoolers when they are in or near water, whether in the tub or in a pool. Schedule baths at times when adults (rather than older children) can supervise.
Falls	Seat children in a high chair for snacks and meals, and use a seat belt. Supervise children so that they do not climb out of or fall from the high chair. Supervise climbing activity. Supervise both outdoor and indoor play.
Car-related	**3. Teach Safety** Be a positive role model by "buckling up" yourself and talking about what you are doing.

What You Can Do to Prevent Injuries to Toddlers and Preschoolers

Injury Risks	Prevention Steps
Burns and House Fires	Teach toddlers the meaning of "hot." Teach preschoolers to give matches they find to grown-ups. Teach preschoolers what to do if their clothing catches fire.
Poisoning	Teach toddlers and preschoolers not to eat any parts of indoor or outdoor plants, unless you say it is okay.
General	Give specific safety instructions: "Don't climb the tree." "Stay inside the fence." Frequently remind toddlers and preschoolers what they should and should not do. Teach toddlers to respond to words like "stop" and "no" that you can use in case of danger. Teach preschoolers to tell an adult if they (or anyone else) are hurt.
Medical Identification Bracelet	A child with a special medical problem should always wear an identification bracelet.

Preventing Injuries to Young School-Age Children

About Young School-Age Children

The world of children five to nine years old includes the school and neighborhood as well as the home. Young school-age children spend a lot of time away from their parents. Playing with other children is very important. Learning new skills—riding a bicycle or scooter—is also important. These children want to show their parents, their friends, and themselves just how much they can do. Although they might "know the rules," they are likely to break those rules to see what happens. This is normal for children as they grow and try to find out more about themselves and the world around them.

Between the ages of five and nine, children grow quickly and learn many new skills. It may be difficult for adults to judge their abilities correctly. In making safety rules, remember that children don't think the same way as adults. For example, children often misjudge how far away a car is and how fast it is going. They sometimes mix up left and right and do not understand many traffic signs. Thus, it may be difficult for them to cross a street or ride a bicycle in the street safely.

Some of the steps that parents and other caregivers can take to prevent injuries to young school-age children are shown in the chart, "What You Can Do to Prevent Injuries to Young School-Age Children." As you read this chart, keep in mind that motor vehicle accidents are the leading cause of injury and death for this age group. Other common injuries result from accidents on bicycles and other riding equipment, near-drowning, falls, and sports activities.

The chart shows you some of the ways you can reduce the risk of injury and death to young school-age children. Use the chart to develop your own injury-prevention plan.

Injury Risks	Prevention Steps
Car-related (passenger and pedestrian)	**1. Remove Dangers** Be sure that children "buckle up" properly for each and every ride. Make sure that children play in areas separated from traffic.
Burns and House Fires	Check your home for fire hazards. (Ask your fire department for help with this.) Install smoke detectors and keep them in working order by testing them and replacing batteries when needed. Set the thermostat on your water heater to 120°F. Keep matches, lighters, and cigarettes out of reach. Buy flame-resistant clothing, especially sleepwear.
Bicycles	Check children's bicycles to make sure the size is appropriate. Be sure that bicycles, scooters, and other riding toys do not have any broken parts. Buy an approved helmet for the child to wear when riding and teach him or her to put it on correctly.
Falls	Check playgrounds to make sure the equipment is in good condition. Soft sand or cedar chips under play equipment make it safer.
Drowning	If you have a home swimming pool, fence it completely around to prevent access from the house by your child.
Bicycles	**2. Give Supervision** Make sure that a child wears a helmet when riding a bicycle.
Drowning	Supervise children's water play.
General	Since you are not always with your children, be familiar with the places they usually go. For instance, you should be familiar with the route to school, the school yard, neighbors' houses, and where your children go after school. Be sure you know how other caregivers supervise your children when you are not there. Make clear the kind of supervision you expect for your children.
Car-related	**3. Teach Safety** Be a positive role model by always "buckling up" yourself.
Bicycles	Teach children safe riding practices such as obeying traffic signs. Stress the importance of not fooling around with other children while riding.

What You Can Do to Prevent Injuries to Young School-Age Children

Injury Risks	Prevention Steps
Sports-related	Teach children how to use sports equipment properly and to always wear the safety equipment needed for a sport.
Medical Information Bracelet	If a child has a special medical problem, he or she should wear an identification bracelet, and the school should know about this special situation.
Drowning	Teach children to swim. Teach water safety, and give specific rules for swimming, boating, etc.
Burns and House Fires	Teach children not to play with matches.
General	Teach children their telephone number, address, and parents' work telephone numbers. Make sure that young school-age children know how to call the emergency number for the EMS system, police, and fire department. Many communities use 911. Discuss safety rules covering your children's environment: in the house, in the yard, crossing the street, going to school. Reinforce the safety education your children's school provides.

Review Questions

Check the best answer or fill in the blanks with the right word(s).

1. Which of the following will help prevent an infant from choking?
    (Check two.)
    ☐ a. Keeping small objects out of an infant's reach
    ☐ b. Allowing an infant to play with older children's toys
    ☐ c. Giving an infant toys that are too large to be swallowed

2. How can you prevent injuries to infants?
    a. Set the thermostat on the water heater to _____ °F.
    b. Install _____ detectors and keep them in working order.
    c. Put barriers at the _____ and bottom of stairs.
    d. Buckle an infant into an approved car safety _____ on each and every ride.

3. How can you prevent injuries to toddlers and preschoolers?
    a. Make sure they play in areas separated from _____.
    b. Put _____ covers on electrical outlets.
    c. Keep _____, lighters, and cigarettes out of their reach.
    d. Put window guards in rooms above the _____ floor.

4. How can you prevent injuries to young school-age children?
    a. Be sure that they "_____ _____" properly for each and every ride.
    b. Check children's _____ and other riding equipment to make sure the size is appropriate.
    c. Make sure a child wears a _____ when riding a bicycle.
    d. Put _____ or cedar chips under play equipment.

Answers

1. You can help prevent an infant from choking by—
   a. **Keeping small objects out of an infant's reach.**
   c. **Giving an infant toys that are too large to be swallowed.**

2. To prevent injuries to infants you can—
   a. Set the thermostat on the water heater to **120°F.**
   b. Install **smoke** detectors and keep them in working order.
   c. Put barriers at the **top** and bottom of stairs.
   d. Buckle an infant into an approved car safety **seat** on each and every ride.

3. You can prevent injuries to toddlers and preschoolers as follows:
   a. Make sure they play in areas separated from **traffic.**
   b. Put **safety** covers on electrical outlets.
   c. Keep **matches,** lighters, and cigarettes out of their reach.
   d. Put window guards in rooms above the **first** floor.

4. You can prevent injuries to young school-age children as follows:
   a. Be sure that they **"buckle up"** properly for each and every ride.
   b. Check children's **bicycles** and other riding equipment to make sure the size is appropriate.
   c. Make sure a child wears a **helmet** when riding a bicycle.
   d. Put **sand** or cedar chips under play equipment.

One Last Word

This chapter has shown you ways you can prevent injuries to children. Immunization protects children against measles, polio, and other diseases. It is just as important to protect children by removing dangers, giving supervision, and teaching safety. You can reduce the risk of injury by making safety an important part of the way you care for children.

A good way to start is by completing the Home Safety Checklist on pages 191 through 193 of this workbook. The checklist will help you identify dangers in your home so you can remove them.

Certainly, the world is full of risks for people of all ages. But by thinking ahead and doing what you can to protect children, you can greatly reduce their risk of injury.

2 How to Deal With an Emergency (Emergency Action Principles)

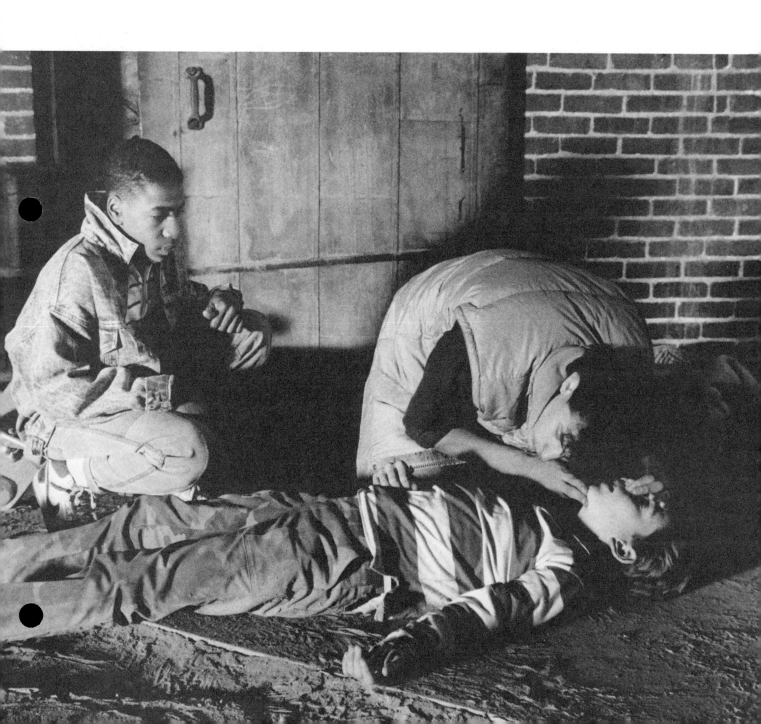

*There are certain steps that you should follow in every emergency. These steps are called the **emergency action principles.** They are discussed in this chapter.*

Objectives

By the time you finish reading this chapter, you should be able to do the following:

1. *List the four emergency action principles (steps you should take in every emergency).*

2. *Explain why you should follow the same steps in every emergency.*

3. *Give two reasons why you should identify yourself as someone trained in first aid before caring for the victim.*

4. *Describe the purpose and steps of a **primary survey.***

5. *Explain why you should finish a primary survey before phoning the emergency medical services (EMS) system for help.*

6. *List at least four important facts you should give an EMS dispatcher when phoning for help.*

7. *Describe the purpose and steps of a **secondary survey.***

8. *Explain when you should get permission before giving first aid to a child or infant.*

Emergency Action Principles

This chapter gives you a four-step plan of action to use in an emergency. In an emergency, you may feel excited, concerned, or scared. A plan of action will help you keep calm so you can help the victim. Following the plan will help keep both you and the victim safe. It will increase the victim's chances of survival. The four steps of the plan are called the **emergency action principles.**

To see why you need to know the emergency action principles, think about this: You are at home watching television when you hear a cry from outside. You run outside and see a child lying facedown on the side of the road. What should you do? Should you phone for an ambulance first? Should you run straight to the child? How could you find out what happened? Once you get to the child, what should you do first? Should you get someone to help you before you go to the child?

Here are the four emergency action principles. Always do the steps in this order. They are explained in this chapter.

1. Survey the scene.
2. Do a primary survey of the victim.
3. Call the emergency medical services (EMS) system for help.
4. Do a secondary survey of the victim.

Review Questions

Fill in the blanks with the right word.

1. Following the emergency action principles will help keep both you and the victim _____.

2. What are the four steps of the emergency action principles?
   a. Survey the _____.
   b. Do a _____ survey.
   c. Phone the _____ system for help.
   d. Do a _____ survey.

Answers

1. Following the emergency action principles will help keep both you and the victim **safe.**

2. The four emergency action principles are—
   a. Survey the **scene.**
   b. Do a **primary** survey.
   c. Phone the **EMS** system for help.
   d. Do a **secondary** survey.

Survey the Scene

When you hear a call for help, the first thing you should do is look around before you go to the victim. This is called surveying the scene. Quickly look all around the victim. This should take only a few seconds. Ask yourself the following questions:

- **Is the scene safe?** Is it safe for you to go to the victim? Look for signs of danger, such as exposed electric wires or passing cars. Once you reach the victim, decide if it is safe for you and the victim to stay where you are. Don't move the victim unless the situation is dangerous.
- **What happened?** Look around for clues. Imagine that you find a half-empty bottle of furniture polish beside an unconscious child. You might guess that the child has swallowed some polish and been poisoned.

  Imagine that you find a child lying next to a bicycle *(Fig. 4).* You would think the child has fallen off the bicycle. The child could have a head injury. It is important to look for clues. An unconscious child or an infant cannot explain what happened or tell you what is wrong.
- **How many people are injured?** Look beyond the victim you see first. There may be other victims. You will notice the child who is screaming in pain. You may not notice another, more seriously hurt child who is unconscious.
- **Are there bystanders who can help?** Look for bystanders— people who are nearby. If a parent or someone else is with an injured child, ask what happened. Try to find out if the child has any medical problems. This information can help you figure out what is wrong with the child. Bystanders can also phone for help. They can take care of any other children who may be at the scene.

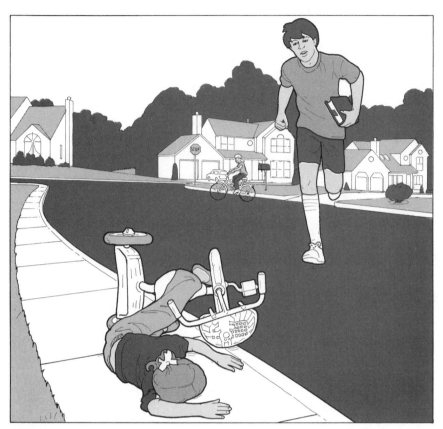

Figure 4
Survey the Scene

Identify Yourself as Someone Trained in First Aid

Tell the victim and bystanders your name. Tell them that you are trained in first aid. This will let other people know you can help. It may also help to reassure the victim.

When an emergency happens in a child-care setting, one person must take charge. Because you are trained in first aid, you should be able to make decisions quickly. Tell other people what they should do to help you, such as phoning for help and caring for other children.

If the child is conscious, tell the child your name if you are a stranger. Tell the child you can help. If the parent or legal guardian of a victim under the age of 18 is there, you should get permission before you give first aid.

If a child or infant is **conscious** but needs first aid right away and the parent or guardian is not there, you should give first aid. You do not need to wait for permission before helping the child. If the child or infant is **unconscious,** you do not need to wait for permission before giving first aid. The parent or guardian's consent is implied. This means that the law assumes that the parent or guardian would have given permission for you to give first aid if they had been present.

Note: The above advice is based on general principles of law. If you want to learn about specific laws where you live, consult an attorney who is qualified to give legal advice in your state or jurisdiction.

Once you reach the injured child or infant, you must find out what's wrong. A child may be able to tell you what happened but may not know all that is wrong. It may be clear that an arm or leg is broken. It may not be so easy to see other injuries. This is why you should follow the same plan of action to find out what is wrong with the victim. Do a primary survey. Next, phone the EMS system for help. Then do a secondary survey.

Review Questions

Check the best answer or fill in the blanks with the right word.

3. What are the four questions you should ask yourself when you survey the scene?
   a. Is the scene _____?
   b. What _____?
   c. How many people are _____?
   d. Are there _____ who can help?

4. Why should you tell the victim and bystanders that you are trained in first aid? (Check two.)
   ☐ a. To learn the names of witnesses
   ☐ b. To reassure the victim
   ☐ c. To let them know you can help

5. A child has fallen off a swing and is sitting on the ground, crying. His parents are kneeling beside him but don't know what to do. What should you do?
   ☐ a. Begin first aid without asking the parents' permission.
   ☐ b. Ask the child where it hurts and phone the EMS system.
   ☐ c. Ask the parents' permission before giving first aid.

6. A child has fallen off a jungle gym in a park. She is lying on the ground, not moving. Some other children are standing around her. What should you do first?
   ☐ a. Begin first aid.
   ☐ b. Send someone to call a doctor.
   ☐ c. Ask the children what happened.

Answers

3. The four questions you should ask yourself when you survey the scene are—
   a. Is the scene **safe?**
   b. What **happened?**
   c. How many people are **injured?**
   d. Are there **bystanders** who can help?

4. You should tell the victim and bystanders that you are trained in first aid in order to—
   b. **Reassure the victim.**
   c. **Let them know you can help.**

5. c. If a child is conscious and his parents are present, you should **ask the parents' permission before giving first aid.**

6. a. You should **begin first aid.** You do not have to wait for permission to help if the child's parent or guardian is not present.

Do a Primary Survey

When you do a primary survey, you look for conditions that are an immediate threat to the victim's life. First, you check for unresponsiveness. You do this to find out if the victim is conscious. Next, you check to see if the victim is breathing and has a pulse.

When you do a primary survey, you check the ABCs—

A—Airway: Does the victim have an open airway (air passage through which the person breathes)?

B—Breathing: Is the victim breathing?

C—Circulation: Is the victim's heart beating? (Does the victim have a pulse?) Is the victim bleeding severely?

Note: Severe bleeding is bleeding that spurts from a wound with every beat of the heart. This bleeding should be controlled **immediately** after checking for a pulse. You can learn how to control bleeding in other American Red Cross first aid courses.

In Chapters 3 and 6 you will learn how to open the airway and check for breathing and circulation. If the child is conscious and is able to talk or is crying, you know the child has an open airway, is breathing, and has a pulse. If you find a problem with the victim's ABCs—**a**irway, **b**reathing, or **c**irculation—you must take care of it right away. Problems with the victim's airway, breathing, or pulse are life-threatening conditions.

Review Questions

Check the best answer or fill in the blanks with the right word.

7. Why do you do a primary survey?
   - [ ] a. To find out what happened to the victim
   - [ ] b. To find conditions that are an immediate threat to the victim's life
   - [ ] c. To find out if the victim has any broken bones

8. When you do a primary survey, which do you do first?
   - [ ] a. Check for bleeding.
   - [ ] b. Check for unresponsiveness.
   - [ ] c. Check for cuts and bruises.

9. When you do a primary survey, you check the victim's ABCs. What do the letters **ABC** stand for?
   A stands for _____.
   B stands for _____.
   C stands for _____.

Answers

7. **b.** You do a primary survey **to find conditions that are an immediate threat to the victim's life.**

8. **b.** When you do a primary survey, the first thing you do is **check for unresponsiveness.**

9. When you do a primary survey, you check the victim's ABCs.
   A stands for **Airway.**
   B stands for **Breathing.**
   C stands for **Circulation.**

Phone the Emergency Medical Services (EMS) System for Help

You should do a primary survey before you phone for help. After you have checked the victim's ABCs, you will know whether the victim is breathing and has a pulse. This information should be given to the EMS dispatcher who answers the phone to help the dispatcher send the right kind of help.

Since you are trained to deal with emergencies, you should stay with the victim, if possible. Send someone else to phone for help *(Fig. 5).* Send two or more bystanders to make the call, if possible. This will make it more likely that the call is made.

When you send someone to call the EMS system, you should do the following:

1. Tell the caller(s) the EMS telephone number. This number is 911 in some communities. If you do not know the special EMS number, tell the caller(s) to dial "0" (the Operator).
2. Tell the caller(s) to give the EMS dispatcher the following important facts:
   - **Where the emergency is.** Give the exact address or location and the name of the city or town. It is helpful to give the names of nearby intersecting streets (cross streets), landmarks, the name of the building, the floor, and the room number.
   - **Telephone number from which the call is being made.**
   - **Caller's name.**
   - **What happened**—choking, car accident, house on fire, etc.
   - **How many people are injured.**
   - **Condition of the victim(s).**
   - **Help (first aid) being given.**
3. Tell the caller(s) not to hang up until the dispatcher hangs up. It is important to make sure the dispatcher has all the information needed to send the right help to the scene.
4. Tell the caller(s) to report back to you after making the call and tell you what the dispatcher said.

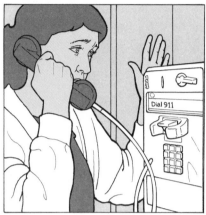

Figure 5
Phone the EMS System

Do a Secondary Survey

The secondary survey is the last step. When you do a secondary survey, you check for injuries or other problems that are not an immediate threat to the victim's life but that could cause problems if not treated. For example, you might find that the child has a broken bone. This is not a life-threatening condition but still should be taken care of.

A secondary survey has three parts:

1. Interview the victim.
2. Check to see if the victim's breathing, pulse, and body temperature are normal.
3. Check the victim from head to toe, looking for injuries.

Interview the Victim

If the child is able to talk, try to find out what is wrong. An older child may be able to tell you what happened.

An injured child or infant is usually frightened. It is very important for you to stay calm. Try not to upset the child or infant even more. When you talk, use a friendly, quiet voice. Say something like, "Hi, my name is _____, and I'm going to help you."

Interview the parents or bystanders. Try to find out the victim's name and age. Does the victim have any medical problems that might have led to the emergency?

The secondary survey is not covered in detail in this course. Most of the emergencies you will learn about in this course are discovered during the primary survey. Other American Red Cross first aid courses deal with the secondary survey. This course focuses on life-threatening conditions that can be found in a primary survey.

Review Questions

Check the best answer and fill in the blanks with the right word.

10. When should you phone the EMS system for help?
  ☐ a. After you have done a primary survey
  ☐ b. After you have found out the victim's name and address
  ☐ c. After you have found out if the victim is unconscious

11. What should you tell the EMS dispatcher when you phone for help?
  a. _____ the emergency is.
  b. _____ number from which the call is being made.
  c. Your _____.
  d. What _____.
  e. How many people are _____.
  f. Condition of the _____.
  g. _____ being given.

12. Why should you do a secondary survey?
  ☐ a. To look for injuries or other problems that are not an immediate threat to the victim's life, but that could cause problems if not treated
  ☐ b. To find out where the victim lives
  ☐ c. To find out what happened

13. What are the three parts of a secondary survey?
  a. Interview the _____.
  b. Check to see if the victim's _____, pulse, and body temperature are normal.
  c. Check the victim from head to toe, looking for _____.

Answers

10. **a.** You should phone the EMS system for help **after you have done a primary survey.**

11. When you phone for help, you should tell the EMS dispatcher—
    a. Where the emergency is.
    b. Telephone number from which the call is being made.
    c. Your **name.**
    d. What **happened.**
    e. How many people are **injured.**
    f. Condition of the **victim(s).**
    g. Help being given.

12. **a.** You should do a secondary survey **to look for injuries or other problems that are not an immediate threat to the victim's life, but that could cause problems if not treated.**

13. The three parts of a secondary survey are—
    a. Interview the **victim.**
    b. Check to see if the victim's **breathing,** pulse, and body temperature are normal.
    c. Check the victim from head to toe, looking for **injuries.**

Summary of Emergency Action Principles

Remember to follow these four steps in every emergency:
1. Survey the scene.
2. Do a primary survey.
3. Phone the EMS system for help.
4. Do a secondary survey.

It is important for you to stay calm and give the right help. If you find a problem during the primary survey, you will have to deal with it at once. For example, if a child is not breathing but has a pulse, you should begin rescue breathing and have someone phone the EMS system for help. In this case, you would not do a secondary survey.

On the other hand, if you do not find any life-threatening problems during the primary survey, you should go on to the secondary survey. For example, if a child has fallen and complains that his leg hurts, you should call the EMS system and begin a secondary survey.

In an emergency it is important for you and your community's EMS system to work together. To learn more about how your EMS system works, read the appendix, "The Emergency Medical Services (EMS) System," on pages 186 through 190 of this workbook. To help you prepare for an emergency, fill out the sheet "Instructions for Emergency Phone Calls," found at the end of this workbook. Post this instruction sheet near a telephone in your home.

3

What to Do When a Child's Breathing Stops (Rescue Breathing)

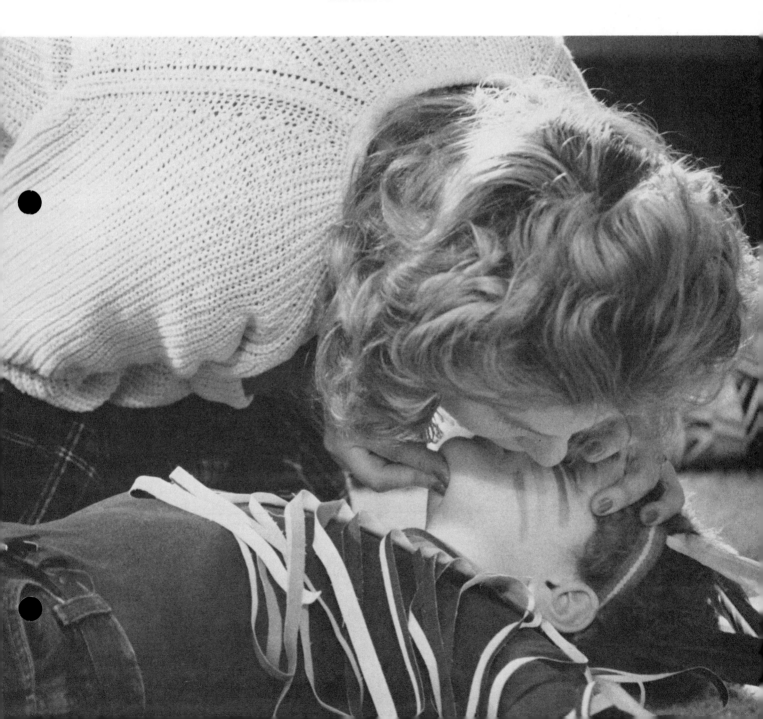

In this chapter, you will learn rescue breathing for a child age one through eight.

Objectives

By the time you finish reading this chapter, you should be able to do the following:

1. *Describe the early signals of a breathing emergency.*
2. *Describe when a child needs rescue breathing.*
3. *Describe how to position a child for rescue breathing.*
4. *Describe how to give rescue breathing to a child.*

Staying Alive

The human body is made of millions of tiny cells. These cells need oxygen to stay alive. Oxygen comes from the air we breathe. Two body systems supply oxygen to the cells: the **respiratory system** and the **circulatory system.**

The **respiratory system** brings oxygen into the body. When we breathe in, air enters the nose and mouth. The air travels down the throat, through the windpipe, and into the lungs. The pathway from the nose and mouth to the lungs is called the **airway.** The airway must be open for air to enter the lungs.

In the lungs the oxygen in the air is picked up by the blood. The blood flows or circulates through the blood vessels, carrying the oxygen to all the cells. The heart pumps the blood through the body. The heart and blood vessels are called the **circulatory system.**

If something blocks the airway, air cannot enter the lungs. Then the blood cannot pick up oxygen. When the cells of the body do not get the oxygen they need, a person dies. Without oxygen, the brain begins to die after four to six minutes.

When a person stops breathing or cannot breathe in enough air to stay alive, a **breathing emergency** occurs. A breathing emergency can lead to a **cardiac emergency** in which the heart stops beating.

Rescue breathing is a way of supplying oxygen to a child whose breathing has stopped. To do rescue breathing, you breathe air from your lungs into the child's lungs. The air you breathe into a child's lungs contains more than enough oxygen to keep the child alive.

Causes and Signals of Breathing Emergencies in Children

A breathing emergency happens when the child's airway becomes blocked in some way. If the airway is blocked, air cannot go through it down into the lungs. There are several ways in which the airway can become blocked.

- **The back of the tongue may drop down into the throat.** This often happens when an unconscious child is lying on his or her back.
- **Tissues in the throat may swell and block the airway.** Swelling may be caused by injuries to the neck. Other causes are burns, allergies, insect stings and bites, and poison. Sometimes an illness may cause the tissues of the throat to swell.
- **An object, such as a piece of food, may block the airway.** The airway may also be blocked by fluids such as vomit or saliva.

Breathing emergencies can also be caused by serious injuries such as electric shock, near-drowning, or injuries from a motor vehicle accident.

It is important to recognize the early signals of a breathing emergency. These signals are often a warning that a breathing emergency is about to happen. Look for any of the following signals:

- Child is agitated or excited.
- Child seems drowsy.
- Child's skin color changes (to pale, blue, or gray).
- Child is having difficulty breathing.
- Child is breathing faster.
- Child's heart is beating faster.

If you believe a child is having a breathing emergency, you should begin first aid. The first aid for a child whose breathing has stopped but whose heart is beating is called rescue breathing.

How to Give Rescue Breathing to a Child

If you find a child lying on the ground and not moving, you should quickly survey the scene and do a primary survey.

1. **Check for Unresponsiveness**
   The first thing you should do is check to see if the child is conscious. Tap or gently shake the child's shoulder. Shout, "Are you OK?" *(Fig. 6)*. Does the child move or make a noise?

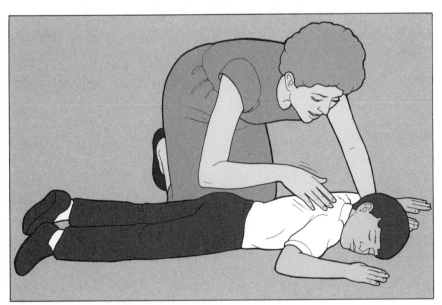

Figure 6
Check for Unresponsiveness

2. **Shout for Help**

   If the child does not move or make a noise, he or she may be unconscious. Shout for help *(Fig. 7)*. Do this to get the attention of people you can ask to phone the EMS system for help after you do a primary survey.

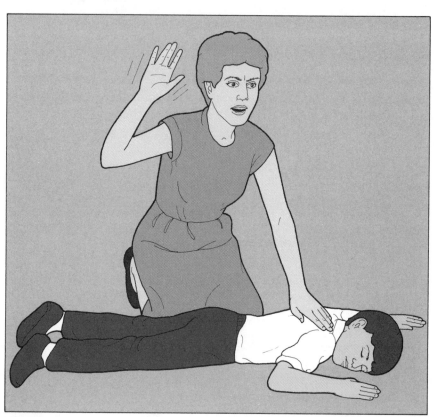

Figure 7
Shout for Help

3. Position the Child

Move the child onto his or her back. To do this, roll the child as a unit *(Fig. 8)*. This will help to avoid twisting the body and making any injuries worse. To position the child—

- Kneel facing the child, midway between the child's hips and shoulders.
- Straighten the child's legs, if necessary.
- Move the child's arm—the one closer to you—so that it is stretched out above the child's head.

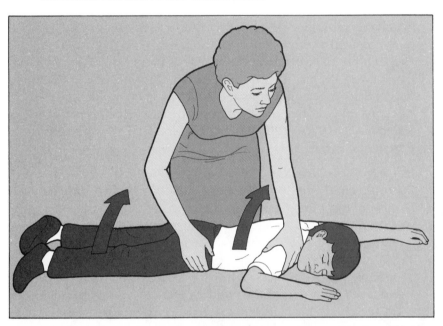

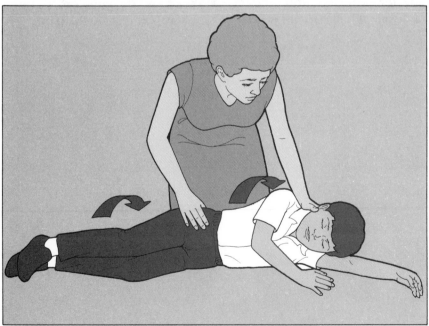

Figure 8
Position the Child

- Lean over the child and place one hand on the child's shoulder. Put your other hand on the child's hip.
- Roll the child toward you as a unit by pulling slowly and evenly. Don't let the child's head and body twist.
- As you roll the child onto his or her back, move your hand from the shoulder to support the back of the head and neck.
- Place the child's arm—the one closer to you—beside the child's body.

It is important to position the child on his or her back as quickly as possible.

Note: Some children who require rescue breathing or CPR may have received a serious injury to the head, neck, or back. Moving these children, or opening the airway as described below, may cause further injury. If you think the child might have a serious head, neck, or back injury, don't move the child. Additional methods for handling these children are discussed in the American Red Cross CPR: Basic Life Support for the Professional Rescuer course.

4. **"A"—Open the Airway**
   Open the child's airway using the **head-tilt/chin-lift** *(Fig. 9)*. This is the most important step you can take to help the child live. To open the airway—
   - Put your hand—the one nearer the child's head—on the child's forehead.
   - Place one or two fingers (not the thumb) of your other hand under the bony part of the child's lower jaw at the chin.
   - Tilt the child's head gently back by applying pressure on the forehead and lifting the chin. Do not close the child's mouth completely. Do not push in on the soft parts under the chin.

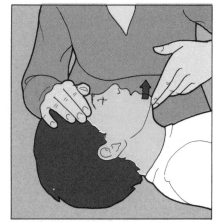

Figure 9
Head-Tilt/Chin-Lift

Tilt the head gently back into the **neutral-plus position.** "Neutral-plus" is a term used to describe the amount of head-tilt necessary to open the airway of a child. A child's airway is different from an adult's or an infant's, and it changes with age. Therefore, there is more than one position for opening the airway. The term "neutral-plus" refers to a range of positions. This range is illustrated in *Figure 10.*

To find the neutral-plus position, begin by tilting the child's head into the neutral position. Remember to lift the chin. Check for breathlessness as described in step 5. Give 2 slow breaths, and watch for the chest to rise and fall, as described in step 6. If the chest does not rise and fall, tilt the head slightly farther back and give 2 slow breaths. Again, watch for the chest to rise and fall.

If necessary, continue tilting the head slightly farther back and giving rescue breaths until the chest rises and falls with each breath.

Once you have found the correct position, take note of it so you can place the child's head in this position each time you give breaths.

Remember: You will know that you have found the correct position when you see the child's chest rise and fall with each breath you give.

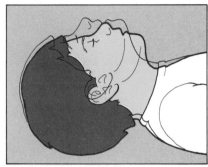

Figure 10
Range of Neutral-Plus Positions

5. **"B"—Check for Breathlessness** (Look, listen, and feel for breathing.)
With the child's head in the neutral-plus position and the chin lifted, check to see if the child is breathing *(Fig. 11).* Tilting the head into the neutral-plus position and lifting the chin opens the airway. This may help the child start breathing again. To check the child's breathing—
- Place your ear just over the child's mouth and nose and look at the child's chest.
- Look, listen, and feel. **Look** for the chest and abdomen to rise and fall. **Listen** for breathing. **Feel** for air coming out of the child's nose and mouth. Do this for 3 to 5 seconds.

If the child is breathing, you will see the chest and abdomen move. You will hear and feel air coming out of the child's nose and mouth. Movement of the chest and abdomen does not always mean that the child is breathing. The child may be trying unsuccessfully to breathe.

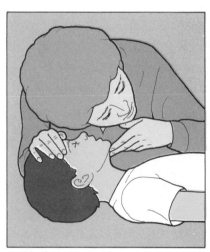

Figure 11
Check for Breathlessness

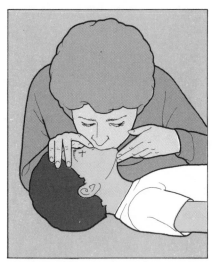

Figure 12
Mouth-to-Mouth Breathing

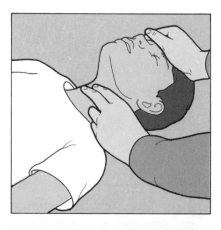

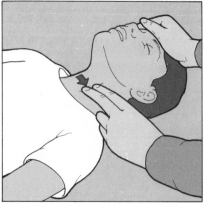

Figure 13
Locate and Feel Carotid Pulse

6. **Give 2 Slow Breaths**

   If the child is not breathing, you must get air into the lungs at once *(Fig. 12)*. To give breaths—
   * Keep the airway open with the head-tilt/chin-lift. Gently pinch the child's nose shut with the thumb and index finger of your hand that is on the child's forehead.
   * Open your mouth wide and take a breath. Seal your lips tightly around the outside of the child's mouth.
   * Give 2 slow breaths. Each breath should last 1 to 1½ seconds. Remove your mouth between breaths just long enough for you to take a breath. Watch for the chest to rise while you breathe into the child. Watch for the chest to fall after each breath. Listen and feel for air coming out of the nose and mouth as the child's chest falls.

   If air will not go in easily, you may not have opened the airway properly. Retilt the child's head and give 2 slow breaths. If air still does not go into the child's lungs, the airway may be blocked by food or some other material. Chapter 4 describes how to help a child whose airway is blocked by food or another object.

7. **"C"—Check Circulation by Checking for a Pulse at the Side of the Neck**

   Check to see if the child's heart is beating by feeling for a pulse at the side of the neck. This pulse is called the **carotid pulse** *(Fig. 13)*. To check for a carotid pulse—
   * Keep one hand on the child's forehead to keep the head in the neutral-plus position. Use your other hand—the one nearer the child's feet—to find the pulse. First, place your index and middle fingers on the child's Adam's apple. Then slide your fingers toward you into the groove between the windpipe and the muscle at the side of the neck. This is where you can feel the child's carotid pulse.
   * Press gently with your fingertips to feel for the beat of the pulse. Be sure to feel for the pulse on the side of the neck closer to you. **Do not use your thumb** because you may feel your own pulse. Feel for the carotid pulse for 5 to 10 seconds.

8. **Phone the EMS System**

   After you have checked the pulse, you will have the information
   the EMS dispatcher needs. Before you send the bystanders to
   phone, tell them whether the child is conscious, breathing, and
   has a pulse. Tell them to give this information to the EMS
   dispatcher.

9. **Begin Rescue Breathing**

   If you feel a pulse and the child is not breathing, then begin rescue
   breathing. (If you do not feel a pulse, the child's heart has stopped.
   You must start CPR, which you will learn in Chapter 5.) To give
   rescue breathing—

   - Keep the child's airway open using the head-tilt/chin-lift.
   - Seal your lips tightly around the child's mouth. Give 1 breath
     every 4 seconds. Each breath should last 1 to 1½ seconds. A
     good way to time the breaths is to count, "One one-thousand,
     two one-thousand, three one-thousand." Take a breath yourself
     and then breathe into the child. Look for the chest to rise as you
     breathe into the child.
   - Between breaths, remove your mouth from the child. Look for
     the chest to fall as you listen and feel at the child's mouth and
     nose for air to come out. Listen to hear if the child starts
     breathing again.

10. **Recheck Pulse**

    After 1 minute of rescue breathing (about 15 breaths), you should check the child's pulse. To check the pulse—
    - Keep the airway open with the hand on the child's forehead.
    - With your other hand feel for the carotid pulse for 5 seconds.

    If the child has a pulse, then check for breathing for 3 to 5 seconds.

    If the child is breathing, keep the airway open. Keep checking breathing and pulse closely. This means that you should look, listen, and feel for breathing. Check the pulse once every minute. Cover the child. Keep the child warm and as quiet as possible.

    If the child is not breathing, continue rescue breathing. Check the pulse once every minute. Continue giving rescue breathing until—
    - The child begins breathing on his or her own.
    - Another trained rescuer takes over for you.
    - EMS personnel arrive and take over.
    - You are too exhausted to continue.

Review Questions

Check the best answer or fill in the blanks with the right word(s).

1. You find a child lying on the ground, not moving. What should you do first?
   - ☐ a. Check the child's pulse.
   - ☐ b. Check for unresponsiveness.
   - ☐ c. Open the airway.

2. How do you open a child's airway?
   - ☐ a. Tilt the head gently back into the neutral-plus position and lift the chin.
   - ☐ b. Put one hand under the child's neck and tilt the head.
   - ☐ c. Push down on the chin.

3. When should you give rescue breathing to a child?
   - ☐ a. When the child is breathing and has a pulse
   - ☐ b. When the child is choking
   - ☐ c. When the child is not breathing but has a pulse

4. How often should you give rescue breaths to a child?
   - ☐ a. Give 1 breath every second.
   - ☐ b. Give 1 breath every 4 seconds.
   - ☐ c. Give 1 breath every 10 seconds.

5. You should continue rescue breathing until one of four things happens. These four things are—
   a. The child starts _____.
   b. Another trained rescuer _____ _____ for you.
   c. _____ personnel arrive and take over.
   d. You are too _____ to continue.

Answers

1. **b.** If you find a child lying on the ground, not moving, the first thing you should do is **check for unresponsiveness.**

2. **a.** To open a child's airway, **tilt the head gently back into the neutral-plus position and lift the chin.**

3. **c.** You should give rescue breathing **when the child is not breathing but has a pulse.**

4. **b.** You should **give a child 1 breath every 4 seconds.**

5. You should continue rescue breathing until one of the following happens:
   a. The child starts **breathing.**
   b. Another trained rescuer **takes over** for you.
   c. **EMS** personnel arrive and take over.
   d. You are too **exhausted** to continue.

More About Rescue Breathing for a Child

Air in the Stomach

Sometimes while doing rescue breathing, you may breathe air into the child's stomach. Air in the stomach can be a serious problem because it makes the stomach swell. Then the lungs do not have enough room to fill with air when rescue breaths are given. Therefore, the child may not get enough oxygen to live.

To keep from forcing air into the child's stomach, do the following:

- **Keep the child's head in the neutral-plus position** to keep the airway open. If you do not see the chest rise and fall with each breath, then tilt the child's head back a little farther and continue rescue breathing.
- **Give slow breaths.** Each breath should last 1 to 1½ seconds.
- **Breathe only enough air to make the chest rise.** Let the chest fall before you give the child another breath.

Vomiting

Sometimes while you are helping an unconscious child, he or she may vomit. It is important that the vomit not get into the lungs. If the child vomits, quickly turn the child's head and body to the side. Wipe out the child's mouth and continue rescue breathing.

Mouth-to-Nose Breathing

There are a few situations in which you may not be able to make a good enough seal over a child's mouth to do rescue breathing. For example, the child's jaw or mouth may have been injured during an accident, or the jaw may be shut too tight to open. In such cases, do mouth-to-nose breathing as follows:

- Put your hand—the one nearer the child's head—on the child's forehead. Remember to tilt the child's head gently back into the neutral-plus position.
- Use your other hand to close the child's mouth by pushing on the chin *(Fig. 14)*. Do not push on the throat.
- Open your mouth wide and take a deep breath. Seal your mouth tightly around the child's nose, and breathe slow breaths into the nose *(Fig. 15)*. Each breath should last 1 to 1½ seconds. If possible, open the child's mouth between breaths by releasing the chin. This will let the air come out *(Fig. 16)*.

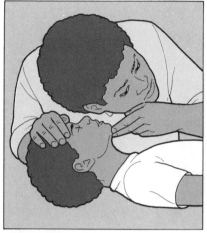

Figure 14
Close Mouth for Mouth-to-Nose Breathing

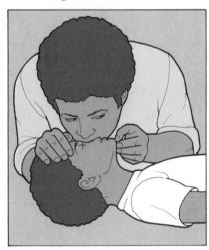

Figure 15
Mouth-to-Nose Breathing

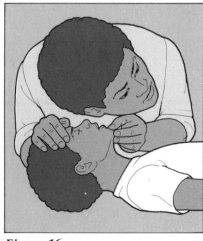

Figure 16
Check for Air Coming Out

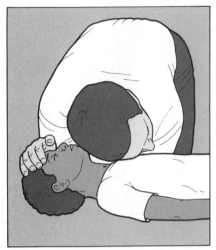

Figure 17
Check Stoma for Breathing

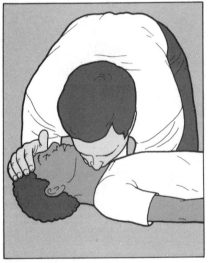

Figure 18
Mouth-to-Stoma Breathing

Mouth-to-Stoma Breathing

There are some children who have had surgery to remove all or part of the upper end of their windpipe. They breathe through an opening called a **stoma** in the front of the neck. This takes the air right into the windpipe, bypassing both the mouth and nose.

Most children who have a stoma wear a bracelet or necklace or carry a card identifying their condition. In an emergency, you may not have time to search for a medical card. It is important to look at the neck area during a primary survey to see if the child has a stoma.

To give rescue breathing to a child with a stoma, you must give breaths through the stoma and not through the mouth or nose. In mouth-to-stoma breathing, you follow the same basic steps as in mouth-to-mouth breathing, except that you—

1. Look, listen, and feel for breathing with your ear held over the stoma *(Fig. 17).*
2. Give breaths into the stoma, breathing at the same rate as for mouth-to-mouth breathing *(Fig. 18).*

There are several other important things you should remember when you give rescue breathing to a child who breathes through a stoma:

- Don't breathe air into the child through the nose or mouth. This may fill the child's stomach with air.
- Never block the stoma since it is the only way the child has to breathe.
- In some cases, a child who has had only part of the upper end of the windpipe removed may breathe through the stoma as well as the nose and mouth. If the child's chest does not rise when you breathe through the stoma, you should close off the mouth and nose and continue breathing through the stoma.

Practice Sessions: Information and Directions

Introduction

In the practice sessions, you will learn how to do rescue breathing, how to help someone who is choking, and how to do CPR (cardiopulmonary resuscitation). You will learn these skills for children and for infants.

During each practice session you will use a skill sheet to help you learn a particular skill. There are directions on the page before each skill sheet. Please read the directions carefully before you start each practice session.

Skill Sheet

The skill sheet contains step-by-step directions on how to practice each skill. There are also pictures to show you what to do. There are two columns of boxes next to the directions. One column is labeled Partner Check. The other is labeled Instructor Check.

Most skill sheets have a section at the end called "What to Do Next." This section will help you decide on the correct first aid if a victim's condition changes.

How to Practice

You will practice each skill in groups of two or three people. You will practice most of the skills on a manikin, taking turns to practice.

One person will be the rescuer and will practice the skills. The second person will act as partner. The partner will read the directions on the skill sheet to the rescuer. If there are three people in your group, the third person will watch to see if the skills are done correctly. After the first rescuer has finished practicing, change places. Each person must practice on the manikin.

You will practice one of the skills on a partner and not on a manikin. When you do this, you will take turns being the victim.

If you need help, ask your instructor.

Directions for the Rescuer

When you begin to practice, have your partner read the skill sheet to you. Your partner should read each step as you practice so you will know what to do.

At some points in the practice, your partner will give you some information about the victim. This is to make the practice seem more like a real emergency. In a real emergency, you would discover this information as you gave first aid.

Practice until you can perform the skills correctly. **Practice** until you feel confident doing the skills. **Practice** until you can perform the skills in the right order, without any directions from your partner. When you can do this, ask your partner to check you.

At the end of most skill sheets is a section called "What to Do Next." Your partner will read this section to you only after you are confident that you know the skill. This section will help you practice changing the care you give if the victim's condition changes. Your partner will give you information about the victim's condition, and you will decide what to do next.

Directions for the Partner

You should read the directions on the skill sheet to the rescuer, step by step. When the rescuer can do the skills correctly without any coaching, begin the Partner Check. When you do the Partner Check, have the rescuer go through the procedure. As the rescuer demonstrates the skill, read the information wherever the skill sheet says, "Partner/Instructor says. . . ." Do not give any other directions unless the rescuer does something wrong. As the rescuer does each step correctly, check the box by that step in the Partner Check column.

When the rescuer can do the entire procedure correctly, read one of the statements in the "What to Do Next" section at the appropriate point in the procedure.

If the rescuer can't go through all the steps correctly, help the rescuer practice some more.

Instructor Skill Test

When all the members of your group have practiced and are ready to be tested, ask the instructor to test your skills. During the skill test, the instructor will ask you to go through all the steps without coaching. When you complete the procedure correctly, the instructor will sign your workbook.

If the instructor sees a serious error, he or she will stop you and correct you. You will be asked to practice some more before being tested again. Ask your partner to work with you. When you have practiced and feel that you are ready to be tested again, ask the instructor to retest you.

Practice on Each Other

You will practice one skill on a partner. By practicing on each other, you will learn how it feels to work on a real person.

When practicing on a partner, follow the skill sheet directions but do not give actual abdominal thrusts.

Practice on a Manikin

Before you practice on the manikin, clean its face and the inside of its mouth. Directions for doing this are given in the section called "Some Health Precautions and Guidelines to Follow During This Course" on pages 3 and 4 of this workbook. **Be sure that the manikin's face and mouth have been cleaned before each new member of your group practices, and whenever you change places and begin to practice on the manikin.**

Because it is important to keep the manikin's face clean, the manikin should always be lying on its back. Do not turn the manikin on its face or side to practice positioning a child or infant. First, practice checking for unresponsiveness. Then go directly to the step, "Open the Airway."

Health Precautions

Before you start practicing, read "Some Health Precautions and Guidelines to Follow During This Course" on pages 3 and 4 of this workbook. If you have any questions or if there is any reason that you should not take part in the practice sessions, it is important that you talk with your instructor.

Practice Session: Rescue Breathing for a Child

During this practice session, you and a partner will practice on a manikin. You will practice all the steps and will give actual rescue breaths.

Before you start practicing, carefully read the skill sheet on pages 59 through 62. If you don't remember how to use the skill sheets, read pages 55 through 57, "Practice Sessions: Information and Directions."

Before you practice on the manikin, clean its face and the inside of its mouth. Directions for doing this are given in the section called "Some Health Precautions and Guidelines to Follow During This Course" on pages 3 and 4 of this workbook. **Clean the manikin's face and mouth before each person in your group practices.**

Skill Sheet: Rescue Breathing for a Child

You find a child lying on the ground, not moving. You should survey the scene to see if it is safe for you to go to the child and to get some idea of what happened. Then do a primary survey.

Partner Check

Instructor Check

☐ ☐ **Check for Unresponsiveness** (Does the child respond?)

Tap or gently shake child's shoulder.

Rescuer shouts, "Are you OK?"

Partner/Instructor says, "Unconscious."

Rescuer repeats, "Unconscious."

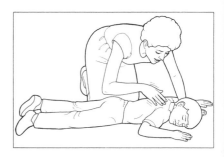

Rescuer shouts, "Help!"

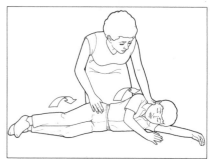

Position the Child

Roll child onto back, if necessary.

Kneel facing child, midway between child's hips and shoulders.

Straighten child's legs, if necessary, and move child's arm—the one closer to you—above child's head.

Lean over child and place one hand on child's shoulder and your other hand on child's hip.

Roll child toward you as a unit. As you roll child, move your hand from shoulder to support back of head and neck.

Put child's arm—the one closer to you—beside child's body.

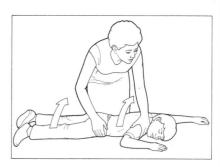

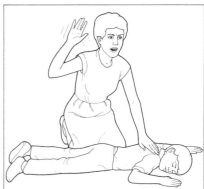

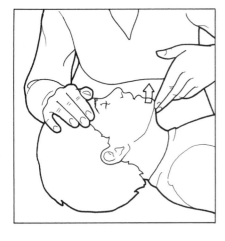

Partner Check
Instructor Check

☐ ☐ **Open the Airway** (Use head-tilt/chin-lift.)

Place your hand—the one nearer the child's head—on the child's forehead.

Put fingers of other hand under bony part of lower jaw at the chin.

Tilt head gently back into the neutral-plus position and lift chin. Do not close child's mouth completely. Do not push on the soft parts under the chin.

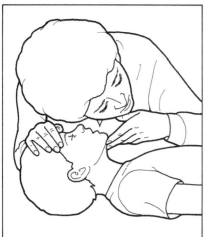

☐ ☐ **Check for Breathlessness** (Is the child breathing?)

Keep airway open with head-tilt/chin-lift.

Place your ear over child's mouth and nose.

Look at chest and abdomen. Listen and feel for breathing for 3 to 5 seconds.

Partner/Instructor says, "No breathing."

Rescuer repeats, "No breathing."

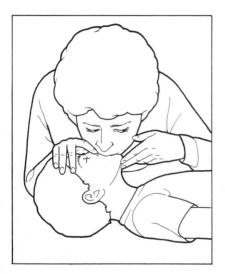

☐ ☐ **Give 2 Slow Breaths**

Keep airway open with head-tilt/chin-lift.

Pinch child's nose shut.

Open your mouth wide and take a breath. Seal your lips tightly around outside of child's mouth.

Give 2 slow breaths. Each breath should last 1 to 1½ seconds. Take a breath yourself between the breaths you give the child.

Look for the chest to rise and fall. Listen and feel for air coming out of the child's nose and mouth.

Partner Check
Instructor Check

☐ ☐ **Check for Pulse**

Keep child's head tilted with one hand on forehead.

Locate Adam's apple with middle and index fingers of hand nearer child's feet.

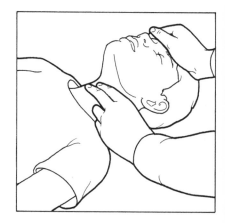

Slide fingers toward you into groove of neck on side closer to you.

Feel for carotid pulse for 5 to 10 seconds.

Partner/Instructor says, "No breathing, but there is a pulse."

Rescuer repeats, "No breathing, but there is a pulse."

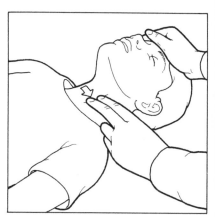

☐ ☐ **Phone the EMS System for Help**

Tell someone to call for an ambulance.

Rescuer says, "Child not breathing, but has a pulse, call _____."

(Local emergency number or Operator)

Partner Check
Instructor Check

☐ ☐ **Now Begin Rescue Breathing**

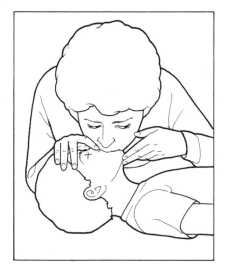

Keep airway open with head-tilt/chin-lift.

Pinch nose shut.

Open your mouth wide and take a breath. Seal your lips tightly around outside of child's mouth.

Give 1 breath every 4 seconds. Each breath should last 1 to 1½ seconds. Count aloud, "One one-thousand, two one-thousand, three one-thousand." Take a breath yourself and then breathe into the child.

Look for the chest to rise and fall. Listen and feel for air coming out of the child's nose and mouth.

Continue for 1 minute—about 15 breaths.

☐ ☐ **Recheck Pulse**

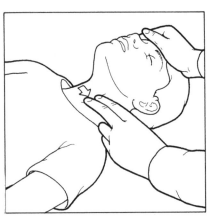

Keep child's head tilted with one hand on forehead.

With other hand feel for carotid pulse for 5 seconds.

Partner/Instructor says, "Has a pulse."

Rescuer repeats, "Has a pulse."

Look, listen, and feel for breathing for 3 to 5 seconds.

Partner/Instructor says, "No breathing."

Rescuer repeats, "No breathing."

☐ ☐ **Continue Rescue Breathing**

Keep airway open with head-tilt/chin-lift.

Give 1 breath every 4 seconds. Each breath should last 1 to 1½ seconds.

Recheck pulse once every minute.

☐ ☐ **What to Do Next**

While the rescuer is rechecking pulse and breathing, the partner should read one of the following statements:

1. Child is breathing but is still unconscious.

2. Child has a pulse but is not breathing.

The rescuer should use this information to decide what to do next and then give the right care.

Final Instructor Check_____

Review Section: Rescue Breathing for a Child

A seven-year-old boy has just been pulled out of a swimming pool. You check for unresponsiveness. He does not respond. He is unconscious. Next, you check the ABCs.

1. What do the letters **ABC** stand for?
   A stands for _____.
   B stands for _____.
   C stands for _____.

   The boy is not breathing but does have a pulse. Someone calls the EMS system while you begin rescue breathing.

2. How often should you give breaths to a child?
   ☐ a. Give 1 breath every second.
   ☐ b. Give 1 breath every 4 seconds.
   ☐ c. Give 1 breath every 8 seconds.

   You recheck the pulse after 1 minute of rescue breathing. The child still has a pulse.

3. What should you do next?
   ☐ a. Check for breathing for 3 to 5 seconds.
   ☐ b. Continue rescue breathing.

4. If the child starts to breathe on his own, what should you do until EMS personnel arrive?
   ☐ a. Leave the child alone.
   ☐ b. Keep the airway open and check breathing and pulse closely.
   ☐ c. Continue giving 1 breath every 4 seconds.

Answers

1. A stands for **Airway.**
   B stands for **Breathing.**
   C stands for **Circulation.**

2. **b.** For a child, you should **give 1 breath every 4 seconds.**

3. **a.** You should **check for breathing for 3 to 5 seconds** if the child has a pulse.

4. **b.** You should **keep the airway open and check breathing and pulse closely** until EMS personnel arrive if the child starts to breathe on his own.

4

What to Do for a Child Who Is Choking

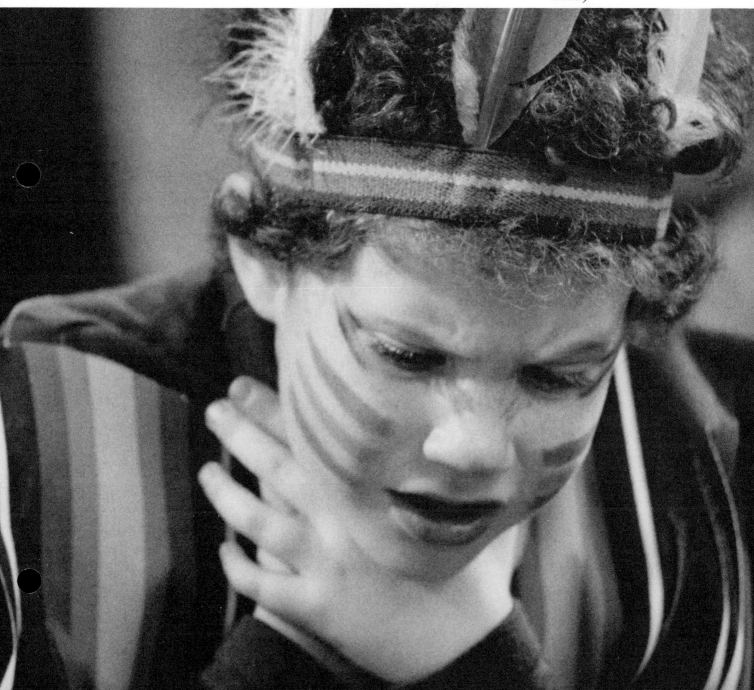

In this chapter, you will learn what to do when a child is choking. When this happens, the child can quickly stop breathing, lose consciousness, and die. You will learn how to tell if a child is choking. You will learn how to tell if the child needs first aid. You will also learn the first aid for choking. A child who is choking has a blocked airway.

Objectives

By the time you finish reading this chapter, you should be able to do the following:

1. *Describe the signals of choking in a conscious child.*
2. *Describe the first aid for a conscious child who is choking.*
3. *Describe how you would find out that an unconscious child has a blocked airway.*
4. *Describe the first aid for an unconscious child with a blocked airway.*
5. *Describe the first aid for a conscious child who becomes unconscious while choking.*

Causes and Signals of Choking

Choking is a common childhood injury that can lead to death. When a child is choking, the airway is partially or completely blocked. Here are some actions that can cause choking:

- **Trying to swallow a piece of food that is poorly chewed.** A child's teeth, mouth, and esophagus are smaller than an adult's. A child can choke on a very small piece of food. Also, children cannot and do not always chew food well. Some foods that an adult can eat easily can cause a child to choke. So, to prevent choking, cut a child's food into small pieces. Do not give a young child nuts, popcorn, and other foods that could get stuck in the airway and cause choking.

- **Talking or laughing while eating, or eating too fast.** To prevent choking, supervise children while they eat. Do not let them eat too fast or get overexcited during a meal or snack.

- **Walking, running, or playing while eating.** To prevent choking, have children sit when they eat. Do not let them move around while eating snacks.

- **Putting an object in the mouth to taste or explore it.** Young children, especially those under the age of three, often put objects such as coins, beads, and toys in their mouth. Tasting is one way children explore their world. It is normal but can lead to choking. To prevent choking, always act when you suspect a child has an object in his or her mouth. Make a toddler spit out the object, or remove the object with your fingers. Regularly check the floors, rugs, and other places for pins, coins, and other small objects that a child might pick up and put in his or her mouth.

A choking child can quickly stop breathing, lose consciousness, and die. Therefore, it is very important to recognize when a child needs first aid for choking. These are signals that a child is choking:

- **The child coughs forcefully.** This can be a signal that the child's airway is partially blocked but that the child is still able to breathe.

  If a child is coughing forcefully, stay with the child. Tell the child to keep on coughing. The coughing may clear the airway. If the child does not stop coughing soon, call the EMS system for help.

- **The child coughs weakly or makes a high-pitched sound** while breathing. These signals mean that a child's airway is partially blocked and that the child cannot breathe properly.

- **The child cannot speak, breathe, or cough.** This means that the child's airway is completely blocked. The child may panic and clutch at his or her throat with one or both hands. This is the universal distress signal for choking *(Fig. 19).*

If a child's airway is partially or completely blocked, and the child cannot breathe properly, you should give first aid to clear the airway.

Review Questions

Check the best answer.

1. A child is choking on a piece of candy. The child is conscious and is coughing forcefully. What should you do?
   - ☐ a. Slap the child on the back.
   - ☐ b. Stay with the child and tell the child to keep on coughing.
   - ☐ c. Give the child a drink of water.

2. A conscious child is choking. The child cannot speak or breathe. What should you do?
   - ☐ a. Give first aid to clear the airway.
   - ☐ b. Watch the child carefully.
   - ☐ c. Slap the child on the back.

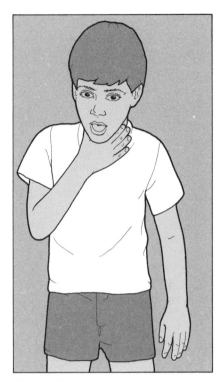

Figure 19
Universal Distress Signal for Choking

Answers

1. **b.** When a conscious child is choking and is coughing forcefully, you should **stay with the child and tell the child to keep on coughing.**

2. **a.** When a conscious child is choking and cannot speak or breathe, you should **give first aid to clear the airway.**

First Aid for Choking (Conscious Child)

You should give first aid for choking if—
- A child cannot cough, speak, or breathe.
- A child is coughing weakly or making high-pitched noises.

If you see a child who is coughing weakly and making high-pitched noises or who is unable to cough, speak, or breathe, you should survey the scene as you approach the child.

1. Begin a primary survey by asking, "Are you choking?"
2. If you are alone, shout for help.
3. Tell the child that you are trained in first aid and can help. Have someone phone the EMS system for help.
4. Do abdominal thrusts (sometimes called the Heimlich maneuver) as follows:
   - Stand or kneel behind the child. The child should be standing or sitting. Wrap your arms around his or her waist. Make a fist with one hand. Place the thumb side of your fist against the middle of the child's abdomen, just above the navel and well below the lower tip of the breastbone *(Figs. 20, 21, and 22)*.

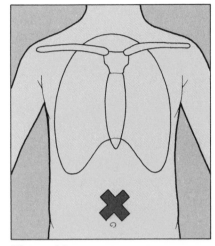

Figure 20
Location for Abdominal Thrusts

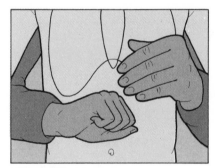

Figure 21
Location for Abdominal Thrusts

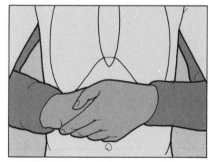

Figure 22
Hand Placement for Abdominal Thrusts

- Grasp your fist with your other hand. Keep your elbows out and away from the child. Be sure that your fist is directly on the midline of the child's abdomen. Press your fist into the child's abdomen with a quick upward thrust *(Fig. 23).* Try to dislodge the object with each thrust.

5. Repeat the thrusts until the airway is clear or until the child becomes unconscious.

Later in this chapter, you will learn how to help a choking child who becomes unconscious.

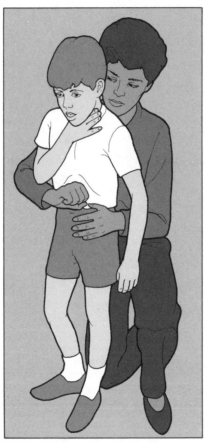
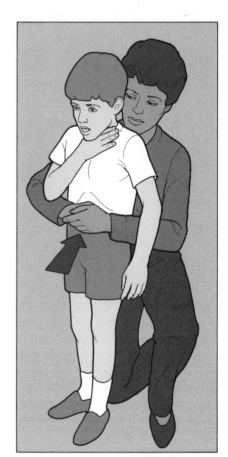

Figure 23
Giving Abdominal Thrusts

When to Stop

Stop giving thrusts as soon as the object is coughed up or the child starts to breathe or cough. Watch the child, and make sure that the child is breathing freely again. Even after the child coughs up the object, the child may have breathing problems that will need a doctor's attention. You should also realize that abdominal thrusts may cause injuries. For these reasons, you should call the EMS system if you have not already done so. **The child should be taken to the hospital emergency department to be checked by a doctor. Do this even if the child seems to be breathing well.**

Review Questions

Check the best answer(s).

3. When should you give abdominal thrusts to a conscious child who is choking? (Check two.)
   - ☐ a. When the child is coughing weakly or making high-pitched noises
   - ☐ b. When the child is coughing forcefully
   - ☐ c. When the child cannot cough, speak, or breathe

4. When you give abdominal thrusts to a conscious child, what position should the child be in?
   - ☐ a. Lying on his or her back
   - ☐ b. Sitting or standing
   - ☐ c. Kneeling down

5. When you give abdominal thrusts to a conscious child, what part of your fist should you place against the child's abdomen?
   - ☐ a. The palm side
   - ☐ b. The thumb side
   - ☐ c. The knuckles

6. When you give abdominal thrusts to a conscious child, where should you place your fist?
   - ☐ a. At the lower tip of the breastbone
   - ☐ b. Just above the navel and well below the lower tip of the breastbone
   - ☐ c. On the navel

7. How should you give abdominal thrusts to a conscious child?
   - ☐ a. Using a quick upward thrust
   - ☐ b. Using a downward thrust
   - ☐ c. Using slow inward pressure

Answers

3. a. You should give abdominal thrusts **when the child is coughing weakly or making high-pitched noises.**

   c. You should give abdominal thrusts **when the child cannot cough, speak, or breathe.**

4. b. When you give abdominal thrusts to a conscious child, the child should be **sitting or standing.**

5. b. When you give abdominal thrusts to a conscious child, you should place **the thumb side** of your fist against the child's abdomen.

6. b. When you give abdominal thrusts to a conscious child, you should place your fist **just above the navel and well below the lower tip of the breastbone.**

7. a. You should give abdominal thrusts to a conscious child **using a quick upward thrust.**

First Aid for Choking (Unconscious Child)

First aid for any unconscious child begins with a primary survey. While checking the ABCs, you may find that the child has a blocked airway. The procedure for finding out if an unconscious child has a blocked airway is given below. First, survey the scene. Then do a primary survey.

1. Check for unresponsiveness.
2. Shout for help.
3. Position the child on his or her back.
4. Open the airway.
5. Look, listen, and feel for breathing for 3 to 5 seconds.
6. If the child is not breathing, give 2 slow breaths.
7. If you are unable to breathe air into the child, retilt the head and give 2 more breaths. You may not have tilted the child's head into the correct position the first time.

If you still cannot breathe air into the child, tell someone to phone the EMS system for help, and do the following:

8. Give 6 to 10 abdominal thrusts (as explained on page 74).
9. Do a foreign-body check (as explained on pages 74 and 75).
10. Open the airway and give 2 slow breaths.

Repeat steps 8, 9, and 10 until the airway is clear or EMS personnel arrive and take over.

Abdominal Thrusts

To give abdominal thrusts to an unconscious child—

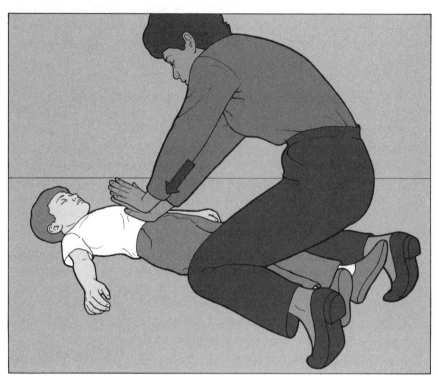

Figure 24
Abdominal Thrusts for Unconscious Child

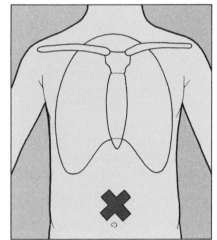

Figure 25
Location for Abdominal Thrusts

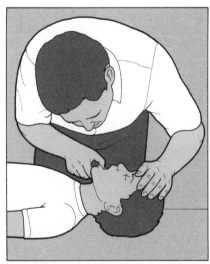

Figure 26
Foreign-Body Check

- Kneel at the child's feet. If the child is large, straddle the child's legs *(Fig. 24)*.
- Place the heel of one hand against the middle of the child's abdomen, just above the navel and well below the lower tip of the breastbone *(Fig. 25)*. Put your other hand on top of your first hand. The fingers of both hands should be pointed toward the child's head. Do not press your fingers on the child's ribs.
- Press into the abdomen with a quick upward thrust. Give 6 to 10 thrusts. Be sure that your hands are directly on the midline of the abdomen when you press. Do not thrust to the right or to the left. Try to dislodge the object with each thrust.
- After you have given 6 to 10 abdominal thrusts, do a foreign-body check to find out if the object has been dislodged.

Foreign-Body Check

To do a foreign-body check—
- Kneel beside the child's head.
- Open the child's mouth using your hand that is nearer the child's feet. Put your thumb into the mouth and grasp both the tongue and the lower jaw between your thumb and fingers. Lift the jaw upward *(Fig. 26)*. This lifts the tongue away from the back of the throat and away from any object that may be lodged there.

- Look for the object. If you can see an object, try to remove it with the finger sweep *(Figs. 27, 28)*.

  To do the finger sweep—
- Slide the little finger of your other hand into the child's mouth. Slide your finger down along the inside of the cheek to the base of the child's tongue. Be careful not to push the object deeper into the airway.
- Use a hooking action to sweep the object out of the throat.

Remember: Do the finger sweep only if you can see the object in the child's throat.

2 Slow Breaths

After you do the foreign-body check, give 2 slow breaths as follows:
- Open the airway with the head-tilt/chin-lift.
- Give 2 slow breaths.

  Continue these three steps:
1. Give 6 to 10 abdominal thrusts.
2. Do a foreign-body check.
3. Open the airway and give 2 slow breaths.

If your first attempts to clear the airway are unsuccessful, do not stop. The longer the child goes without oxygen, the more the muscles of the throat will relax. This will make it more likely that you will be able to remove the object.

If you do clear the airway and can breathe into the child, give 2 slow breaths as you did for rescue breathing. Then check the child's pulse. If there is no pulse, begin CPR. You will learn how to do CPR for a child in Chapter 5. If there is a pulse, check for breathing. If the child is not breathing on his or her own, continue rescue breathing.

If the child starts breathing on his or her own, keep checking the child's breathing and pulse until EMS personnel arrive and take over. This means you should keep the airway open. Look, listen, and feel for breathing. Keep checking the pulse. Cover the child. Keep the child warm and as quiet as possible.

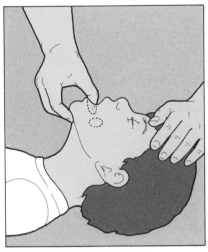

Figure 27
Grasp Tongue and Lower Jaw

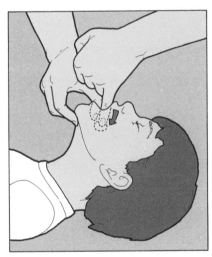

Figure 28
Finger Sweep for a Child

Put the Steps Together

Here are the steps for helping an unconscious child whose airway may be blocked:

1. Check for unresponsiveness.
2. Shout for help.
3. Position the child on his or her back.
4. Open the airway.
5. Look, listen, and feel for breathing for 3 to 5 seconds.
6. If the child is not breathing, give 2 slow breaths.
7. Retilt the head if you cannot breathe air into the child.
8. Give 2 slow breaths.

If you are still unable to breathe air into the child's lungs, have someone phone the EMS system for help and—

9. Give 6 to 10 abdominal thrusts.
10. Do a foreign-body check.
11. Open the airway and give 2 slow breaths.

Repeat steps 9, 10, and 11 until the airway is clear or EMS personnel arrive and take over. If you succeed in removing the object, open the airway and give 2 slow breaths. Then check for a pulse. If there is no pulse, begin CPR. If there is a pulse, check for breathing. If the child is not breathing on his or her own, continue rescue breathing.

Review Questions

Check the best answer.

8. A child is unconscious and is not breathing. You cannot breathe air into the child's lungs when you give the first 2 breaths. What should you do next?
   - [ ] a. Retilt the child's head and give 2 more breaths.
   - [ ] b. Look in the mouth for an object blocking the airway.
   - [ ] c. Give 6 to 10 abdominal thrusts.

9. You are giving abdominal thrusts to an unconscious child. Where should you kneel?
   - [ ] a. Kneel by the child's chest.
   - [ ] b. Kneel by the child's head.
   - [ ] c. Kneel at the child's feet or straddle the child's legs.

10. You are giving abdominal thrusts to an unconscious child. Where should you place your hands?
    - [ ] a. Over the edge of the rib cage
    - [ ] b. Against the middle of the child's abdomen, just above the navel and well below the lower tip of the breastbone
    - [ ] c. Directly over the navel

11. How many abdominal thrusts should you give to an unconscious child before doing a foreign-body check?
    - [ ] a. 1 to 3
    - [ ] b. 6 to 10
    - [ ] c. 15 to 20

12. After you remove an object from a child's mouth, you give the child 2 breaths and see the chest rise and fall. What should you do next?
    - [ ] a. Open the airway.
    - [ ] b. Check the pulse.
    - [ ] c. Phone the EMS system for help.

Answers

8 a. You should **retilt the child's head and give 2 more breaths** if you cannot breathe air into the lungs of an unconscious child who is not breathing.

9. c. When you are giving abdominal thrusts to an unconscious child, you should **kneel at the child's feet or straddle the child's legs.**

10. b. When you are giving abdominal thrusts to an unconscious child, you should place your hands **against the middle of the child's abdomen, just above the navel and well below the lower tip of the breastbone.**

11. b. You should give **6 to 10** abdominal thrusts to an unconscious child before doing a foreign-body check.

12. b. When you can breathe into the child, the next thing you should do is **check the pulse.**

First Aid for Choking When a Conscious Child Becomes Unconscious

Sometimes a choking child may lose consciousness. If this happens, you should shout for help. Slowly lower the child to the floor while you support the child from behind. Support the child's head as you lower the child to the floor.

Once the child is on the floor, tell someone to phone the EMS system for help if it hasn't already been done. Then kneel beside the child and do the following:

1. Do a foreign-body check.
2. Open the airway and give 2 slow breaths.
3. Give 6 to 10 abdominal thrusts if you are unable to breathe into the child's lungs.

Repeat these three steps until the airway is clear or EMS personnel arrive and take over.

Practice Sessions: First Aid for Choking

First, you will learn first aid for a conscious child with a blocked airway. Later on, you will learn first aid for an unconscious child with a blocked airway.

Practice Session 1: First Aid for Choking (Conscious Child)
You will learn the first aid for a conscious child with a blocked airway. You will practice this skill on a partner. The instructor will read the directions out loud as you practice.

Remember: **When practicing abdominal thrusts on a partner, do not give actual abdominal thrusts.**

Practice Session 2: First Aid for Choking (Unconscious Child)
You will learn the first aid for an unconscious child with a blocked airway. You will practice this skill on a manikin. Before you start practicing, carefully read the following directions and the skill sheet on pages 82 through 86. If you don't remember how to use the skill sheet, read "Practice Sessions: Information and Directions" on pages 55 through 57.

Remember: **Do not touch the manikin's lips or inside the mouth with your fingers.**

Before you practice on the manikin, clean its face and the inside of its mouth. Directions for doing this are given in the section called "Some Health Precautions and Guidelines to Follow During This Course" on pages 3 and 4 of this workbook. **Clean the manikin's face and mouth before each person in your group practices.**

Skill Sheet: First Aid for Choking (Conscious Child)

Remember: **While practicing abdominal thrusts, pretend to give thrusts. Never give abdominal thrusts to a person who is not choking.**

Instructor Check

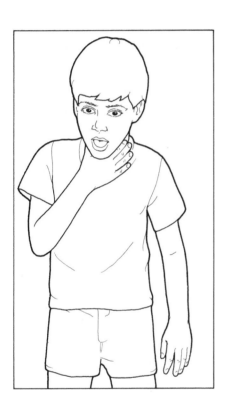

☐ **Find Out if Child Is Choking**

Rescuer asks, "Are you choking?"

Partner/Instructor says, "Child cannot cough, speak, or breathe."

Rescuer shouts, "Help!"

☐ **Phone the EMS System for Help**

Tell someone to call for an ambulance.

Rescuer says, "Child choking, call _____."

(Local emergency number or Operator)

☐ **Do Abdominal Thrusts**

Stand or kneel behind child.

Wrap arms around child's waist.

Make a fist with one hand and put thumb side of fist against middle of child's abdomen, just above navel and well below lower tip of breastbone.

Grasp your fist with your other hand.

Keeping elbows out and away from child, press fist into child's abdomen with a quick upward thrust.

Try to dislodge the object with each thrust.

Repeat thrusts until the airway is clear or child becomes unconscious.

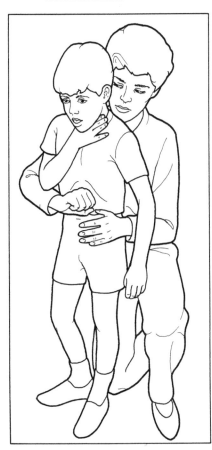
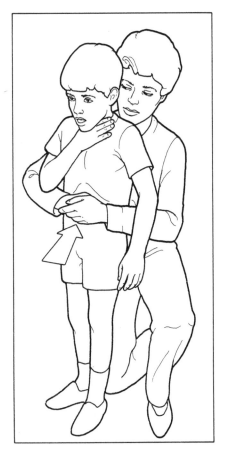

Final Instructor Check_____

Skill Sheet: First Aid for Choking (Unconscious Child)

You find a child lying on the ground, not moving. You should survey the scene to see if it is safe and to get some idea of what happened. Then do a primary survey.

Remember: **Do not do finger sweeps on a manikin. Do not touch the manikin's lips or inside the mouth with your fingers.**

Partner Check
Instructor Check

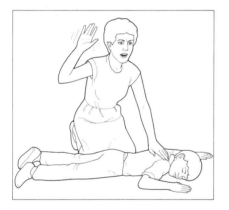

☐ ☐ **Check for Unresponsiveness** (Does the child respond?)

Tap or gently shake child's shoulder.

Rescuer shouts, "Are you OK?"

Partner/Instructor says, "Unconscious."

Rescuer repeats, "Unconscious."

Rescuer shouts, "Help!"

Position the Child

Place the child on his or her back.

☐ ☐ **Open the Airway** (Use head-tilt/chin-lift.)

Place your hand—the one nearer the child's head—on the child's forehead.

Put fingers of other hand under bony part of lower jaw at the chin.

Tilt head gently back into the neutral-plus position and lift chin. Do not close child's mouth completely. Do not push on the soft parts under the chin.

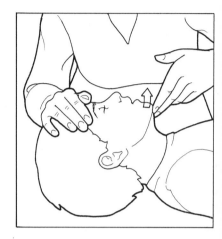

☐ ☐ **Check for Breathlessness** (Is the child breathing?)

Keep airway open with head-tilt/chin-lift.

Place your ear over child's mouth and nose.

Look at chest and abdomen. Listen and feel for breathing for 3 to 5 seconds.

Partner/Instructor says, "No breathing."

Rescuer repeats, "No breathing."

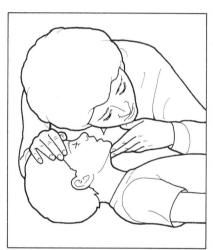

Partner Check
Instructor Check

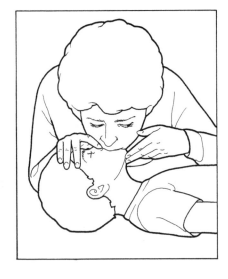

☐ ☐ **Give 2 Slow Breaths**

Keep airway open with head-tilt/chin-lift.

Pinch child's nose shut.

Open your mouth wide and take a breath. Seal your lips tightly around outside of child's mouth.

Give 2 slow breaths. Each breath should last 1 to 1½ seconds. Take a breath yourself between the breaths you give the child.

Partner/Instructor says, "Unable to breathe air into child."

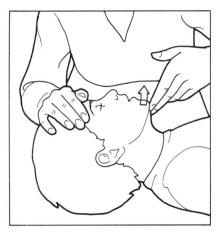

☐ ☐ **Retilt Child's Head and Give 2 Slow Breaths**

Retilt child's head and lift chin. Do not close child's mouth completely. Do not push on the soft parts under the chin.

Pinch child's nose shut.

Open your mouth wide and take a breath. Seal your lips tightly around outside of child's mouth.

Give 2 slow breaths. Each breath should last 1 to 1½ seconds. Take a breath yourself between the breaths you give the child.

Partner/Instructor says, "Still unable to breathe air into child."

Rescuer says, "Airway blocked."

☐ ☐ **Phone the EMS System for Help**

Tell someone to call for an ambulance.

Rescuer says, "Child's airway blocked, call _____."
(Local emergency number or Operator)

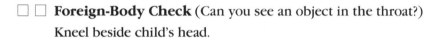

Partner Check
Instructor Check

☐ ☐ **Do 6 to 10 Abdominal Thrusts**

Leave child faceup on his or her back.

Kneel at child's feet or straddle the child's legs.

Locate child's navel.

Place heel of one hand on middle of child's abdomen, just above navel and well below the lower tip of the breastbone.

Place other hand directly on top of first hand. (Fingers of both hands should be pointing toward child's head.)

Press into child's abdomen 6 to 10 times with quick upward thrusts. Try to dislodge the object with each thrust.

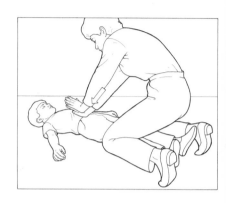

☐ ☐ **Foreign-Body Check** (Can you see an object in the throat?)

Kneel beside child's head.

Open child's mouth and grasp both tongue and lower jaw between thumb and fingers of hand nearer child's legs. Lift jaw.

Look inside mouth for object. If you can see an object, try to remove it with a finger sweep.

Partner/Instructor says, "No object seen."

Rescuer repeats, "No object seen."

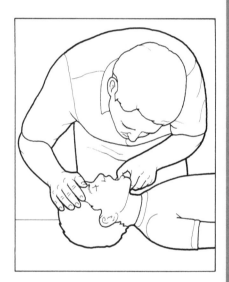

☐ ☐ **Give 2 Slow Breaths**

Keep airway open with head-tilt/chin-lift.

Pinch child's nose shut.

Open your mouth wide and take a breath. Seal your lips tightly around outside of child's mouth.

Give 2 slow breaths. Each breath should last 1 to 1½ seconds. Take a breath yourself between the breaths you give the child.

Partner/Instructor says, "Airway still blocked."

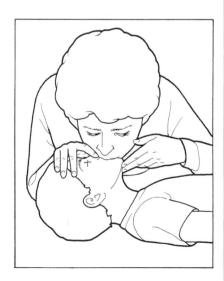

Partner Check
Instructor Check

☐ ☐ **Repeat Sequence**

Do 6 to 10 abdominal thrusts.

Do a foreign-body check.

Give 2 slow breaths.

☐ ☐ **What to Do Next**

While the rescuer is repeating the sequence of abdominal thrusts, foreign-body check, and rescue breaths, the partner should read one of the following statements:

1. Rescuer can breathe into child's lungs after doing foreign-body check.
2. After foreign-body check, object is removed with finger sweep.
3. Object is expelled during abdominal thrusts.

The rescuer should use this information to decide what to do next and then give the right care.

Final Instructor Check_____

Review Section: First Aid for Choking (Conscious Child)

Your five-year-old nephew is eating a piece of hard candy and talking at the same time. Suddenly he stops talking and gags. You ask, "Are you choking?" He cannot speak and grabs his throat. You shout for help and have someone phone the EMS system.

1. Then you give first aid. What is the first aid for a conscious child who is choking?
   ☐ a. Rescue breathing
   ☐ b. Abdominal thrusts
   ☐ c. CPR

2. Which part of your fist should you place against the child's abdomen?
   ☐ a. The thumb side
   ☐ b. Your knuckles

3. When you give abdominal thrusts to a conscious child, where should you place your fist?
   ☐ a. At the lower tip of the breastbone
   ☐ b. Just above the navel and well below the lower tip of the breastbone
   ☐ c. On the navel

4. How should you give abdominal thrusts to a child?
   ☐ a. Using a quick upward thrust
   ☐ b. Using a downward thrust
   ☐ c. Using slow inward pressure

Answers

1. **b.** The first aid for a conscious child who is choking is **abdominal thrusts.**

2. **a.** You should place **the thumb side** of your fist against the child's abdomen when giving abdominal thrusts.

3. **b.** When you give abdominal thrusts to a conscious child, you should place your fist **just above the navel and well below the lower tip of the breastbone.**

4. **a.** You should give abdominal thrusts to a conscious child **using a quick upward thrust.**

Review Section: First Aid for Choking (Unconscious Child)

Your neighbor's child is playing on her swing. She is eating a snack. A few minutes later, you see her lying on the ground. You check for unresponsiveness. She is unconscious.

1. What should you do next?
   - ☐ a. Open the airway.
   - ☐ b. Check for a pulse.
   - ☐ c. Call the EMS system.

2. The child is not breathing, so you give 2 slow breaths. The air will not go in. What should you do now?
   - ☐ a. Do a foreign-body check.
   - ☐ b. Retilt the head and give 2 slow breaths.
   - ☐ c. Begin CPR.

   The air still will not go in. You realize that her airway is blocked. You tell someone to phone the EMS system for help, and then you give abdominal thrusts.

3. How many abdominal thrusts should you give before you do a foreign-body check?
   - ☐ a. 1 to 3
   - ☐ b. 6 to 10
   - ☐ c. 15 to 20

4. After doing the foreign-body check, you should give _____ slow breaths.

Answers

1. **a.** If you find that a child is unconscious, you should **open the airway.**

2. **b.** You should **retilt the head and give 2 slow breaths** if air will not go into the child's lungs.

3. **b.** You should give **6 to 10** abdominal thrusts before you do a foreign-body check.

4. You should give **2** slow breaths after doing the foreign-body check.

5

What to Do When a Child's Heart Stops (CPR)

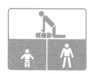

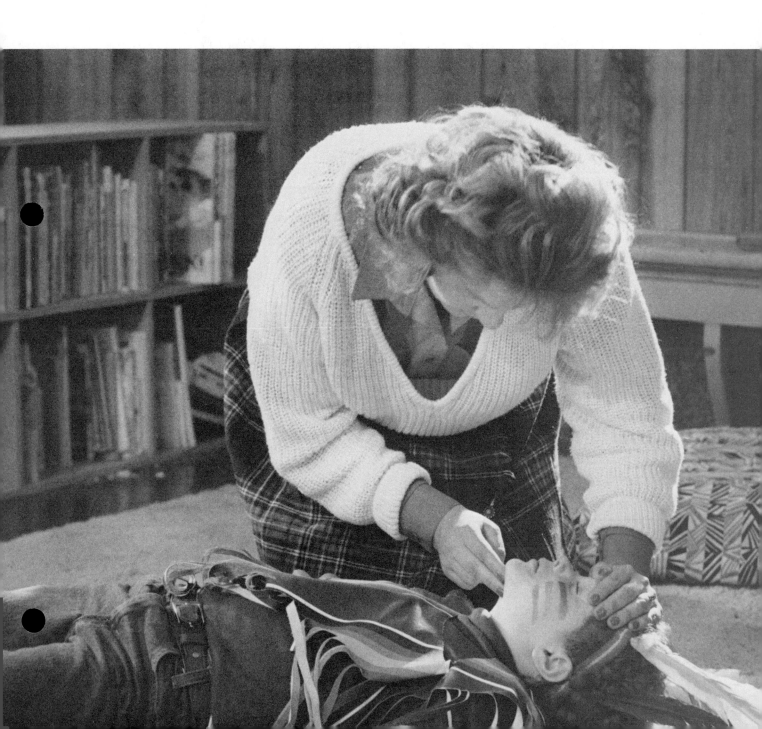

In this chapter, you will learn how to give CPR to a child age one through eight. When a child's heart stops, his or her life depends on how fast CPR is started and how quickly advanced emergency medical help is given.

In this chapter, you will learn what to do for a child whose heart has stopped beating. You will learn how to keep oxygen-carrying blood moving through the child's body.

Objectives

By the time you finish reading this chapter, you should be able to do the following:

1. Describe when a child needs CPR.
2. Explain why you must check the child's carotid pulse before you start CPR.
3. Describe how to give CPR to a child.
4. Explain when you should check to find out if the child's heart is beating again after you have started CPR.
5. List four conditions when a rescuer may stop CPR.

A Look at the Heart

The heart is a tough muscular organ. It is located roughly in the center of the chest between the lungs and under the lower half of the breastbone. The ribs and breastbone protect the heart in the front. The backbone protects the heart in the rear.

The heart pumps blood to all parts of the body through the blood vessels. Blood vessels are the tubes that carry blood to the cells of the body. Blood supplies the oxygen the cells need. If the heart stops beating, it stops pumping blood. Then the cells of the body begin to die.

When a child's heart stops beating, this is a cardiac emergency. The child needs help immediately. CPR helps the child by keeping blood flowing through the body until EMS personnel arrive. To give the child the best chance to live, CPR must be started at once. Advanced emergency medical care must be started within 10 minutes.

The Purpose of CPR and Why It Works

CPR stands for **cardiopulmonary resuscitation.** "Cardio" refers to the heart, and "pulmonary" refers to the lungs. CPR has two parts. One part is chest compressions. When you give chest compressions, you press down and let up on the lower half of the breastbone. The second part of CPR is rescue breaths. Rescue breathing was explained in Chapter 3 of this workbook. When you give CPR, you alternate chest compressions and rescue breaths.

When you breathe into the lungs of a child who has stopped breathing, you keep the lungs supplied with oxygen. The oxygen in the lungs goes into the blood. When you compress the chest, you keep blood flowing through the child's body. The blood carries oxygen to the brain, heart, and other parts of the body. CPR does not restart the heart. It keeps oxygen-carrying blood flowing through the body.

You must start CPR as soon as possible after the child's heart stops beating. If brain cells don't get oxygen, they begin to die after four to six minutes. Starting CPR right away increases the chances that EMS personnel will be able to restart the child's heart.

Review Questions

Fill in the blanks with the right word.

1. The two parts of CPR are chest _____ and rescue _____.

2. CPR supplies oxygen to all parts of the _____.

Answers

1. The two parts of CPR are chest **compressions** and rescue **breaths.**

2. CPR supplies oxygen to all parts of the **body.**

Cardiac Emergencies in Children

Children's hearts are usually healthy. When a child's heart stops, it is usually the result of a breathing emergency. If the child cannot breathe properly, not enough oxygen gets into the blood. This causes the heart to stop beating.

The most common cause of cardiac emergencies in children is injury from motor vehicle accidents. Other injuries that can cause a cardiac emergency are burns, poisoning, near-drowning, and electric shock. A cardiac emergency can happen when a child's airway is blocked. Sometimes a medical condition or an illness, such as severe croup, can cause a cardiac emergency.

Most cardiac emergencies in children can be prevented. One way is to keep children from being injured. Chapter 1 of this workbook describes many ways you can reduce the risk of injury. A second way to prevent cardiac emergencies is to make sure children have proper medical care. A third way is by learning to recognize the early signals of a breathing emergency.

If a breathing emergency is not recognized and treated, a child's heart may stop beating. The following signals are warnings that a breathing emergency may be about to happen:
- Child is agitated or excited.
- Child is drowsy.
- Child's skin color changes (to pale, blue, or gray).
- Child is having difficulty breathing.
- Child is breathing faster.
- Child's heart is beating faster.

In this chapter, you will learn how to help a child whose heart has stopped beating. When a child's heart stops, you must give first aid right away. You must begin CPR to keep oxygen-carrying blood flowing through the body.

How to Give CPR to a Child

Decide if the Child Needs CPR

To find out if a child needs CPR, start with a primary survey. You should—

1. Check for unresponsiveness.
2. Shout for help.
3. Position the child on his or her back.
4. Open the airway.
5. Look, listen, and feel for breathing for 3 to 5 seconds.
6. If the child is not breathing, give 2 slow breaths.
7. Check the carotid pulse for heartbeat for 5 to 10 seconds.
8. Have someone phone the EMS system for help.

If the child has no pulse, begin CPR. **It is important to check the child's carotid pulse for 5 to 10 seconds before you start CPR. It is dangerous to do chest compressions if the child's heart is beating.**

Position Yourself and the Child

Both you and the child must be in the correct position for CPR to work.

To position the child—
* Lay the child on his or her back on a firm, flat surface. The child's head should be on the same level as the heart.

To position yourself—
* Kneel beside the child's chest with your knees against the child's side.
* Use your hand—the one nearer the child's head—to hold the head in the neutral-plus position.

Now find the compression position—
* Use your other hand to find the lower edge of the rib cage on the side closer to you. Slide your middle finger up the edge of the rib cage to the notch where the ribs meet the breastbone in the center of the lower part of the chest *(Figs. 29, 30)*. Put your middle finger in this notch, with the index finger beside it *(Fig. 31)*. The two fingers should be resting on the lower end of the breastbone.

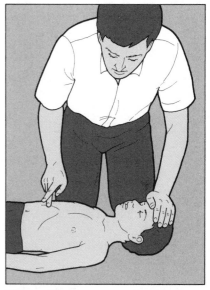

Figure 29
Slide Finger up Edge of Rib Cage

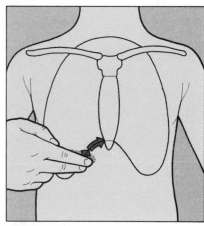

Figure 30
Find Correct Position

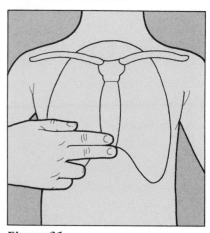

Figure 31
Position Fingers on Breastbone

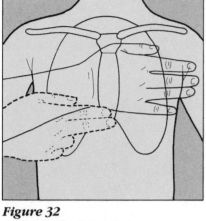

Figure 32
Place Heel of Hand on Breastbone

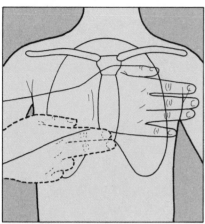

Figure 33
Keep Fingers off Chest

- Look where you put your index finger. Lift your fingers off the breastbone. Put the heel of your hand on the breastbone just above where you had your index finger *(Fig. 32)*.
- Keep your fingers off the child's chest. Only the heel of your hand should rest on the breastbone *(Fig. 33)*. If you have your hand in the correct position, you are less likely to injure the child's ribs or organs when you compress the chest.

- Move your body until your shoulder is directly over your hand *(Fig. 34).*

Give Chest Compressions

1. Use only one hand. Push straight down. Don't rock back and forth *(Fig. 35).*

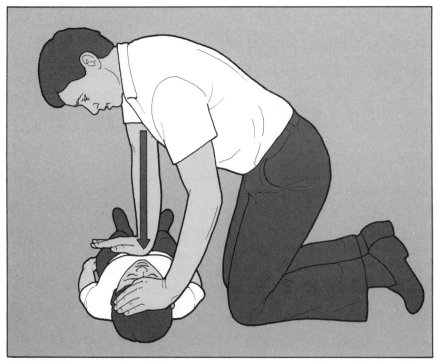

Figure 35
Giving Chest Compressions

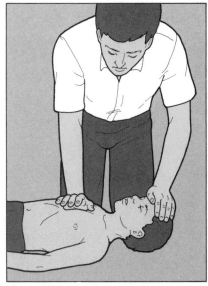

Figure 34
Correct Position of Rescuer

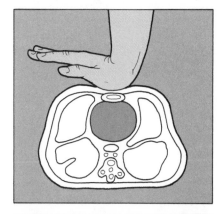

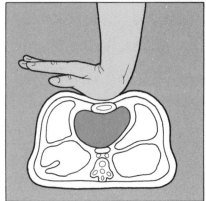

Figure 36
Compress Chest 1 to 1½ Inches

2. Each time you compress, push the child's breastbone down from 1 to 1½ inches (2.5 to 3.8 centimeters) *(Fig. 36).* Then release pressure.
3. Give smooth compressions. Keep a steady down-and-up pace. Do not jerk down and up. Do not pause between compressions. When you come up, release pressure but keep your hand on the chest in the compression position.
4. Give compressions at the rate of 80 to 100 compressions per minute.
5. Look at the correct hand position for compressions. You need to remember it because you have to remove your hand to lift the child's chin and give a breath. Then, you need to return your hand to the correct position before you give compressions again.

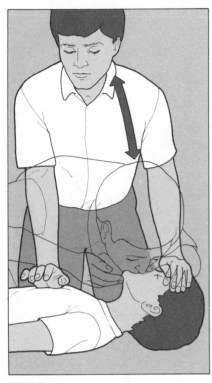

Figure 37
5 Compressions, Then 1 Breath

6. Do cycles of 5 compressions and 1 breath. Count out loud, "One and two and three and four and five and." Push down as you say the number and come up as you say the "and." Do compressions with one hand and keep your other hand on the child's forehead to keep the head in the neutral-plus position *(Fig. 37)*.

   When you give the breath, remove your hand from the chest and lift the chin. Give 1 slow breath. After you give the breath, put your hand back on the child's chest in the correct position for compressions.

7. If your hand moves out of position while you are giving compressions, put it back in place before you continue compressions.

Review Questions

Check the best answer.

3. How should you find the correct hand position to give chest compressions to a child?
   - ☐ a. Slide your middle finger up the edge of the rib cage to the notch where the ribs meet the breastbone.
   - ☐ b. Find the top of the breastbone.
   - ☐ c. Find the navel.

4. When your hand is in place to give compressions, where should your fingers be?
   - ☐ a. Resting on the child's chest
   - ☐ b. Held off the child's chest
   - ☐ c. Curling into your palm

5. While you are giving chest compressions to a child, where should your other hand be?
   - ☐ a. Under the child's shoulders
   - ☐ b. Under the child's head and neck
   - ☐ c. On the child's forehead, keeping the head in the neutral-plus position

6. How far should you compress a child's chest?
   - ☐ a. ½ to 1 inch (1.25 to 2.5 centimeters)
   - ☐ b. 1 to 1½ inches (2.5 to 3.8 centimeters)
   - ☐ c. 1½ to 2 inches (3.8 to 5 centimeters)

7. When you give CPR to a child, at what rate should you give chest compressions?
   - ☐ a. 50 to 60 times per minute
   - ☐ b. 60 to 80 times per minute
   - ☐ c. 80 to 100 times per minute

8. If your hand moves out of place while you are giving chest compressions, what should you do?
   - ☐ a. Put your hand back in place before continuing compressions.
   - ☐ b. Keep on giving compressions.
   - ☐ c. Give a breath before you start compressions again.

Answers

3. a. To find the correct hand position for chest compressions on a child, **slide your middle finger up the edge of the rib cage to the notch where the ribs meet the breastbone.**

4. b. When your hand is in place for compressions, your fingers should be **held off the child's chest.**

5. c. While you are giving compressions to a child, your other hand should be **on the child's forehead, keeping the head in the neutral-plus position.**

6. b. You should compress the chest of a child **1 to 1½ inches (2.5 to 3.8 centimeters).**

7. c. When you give CPR to a child, you should compress the chest at the rate of **80 to 100 times per minute.**

8. a. If your hand moves out of place, **put your hand back in place before continuing compressions.**

Put the Steps Together

Here are the steps for giving CPR to a child:

1. Check for unresponsiveness.
2. Shout for help.
3. Position the child on his or her back on a firm, flat surface.
4. Open the airway.
5. Look, listen, and feel for breathing for 3 to 5 seconds.
6. If the child is not breathing, give 2 slow breaths.
7. Check the child's carotid pulse for heartbeat for 5 to 10 seconds.
8. Tell someone to phone the EMS system for help.
9. If there is no pulse, locate the correct hand position, and position yourself to give chest compressions.
10. Give 5 compressions without stopping, at the rate of 80 to 100 compressions per minute. Keep your other hand on the child's forehead to keep the head in the neutral-plus position.
11. Next, lift the chin, and give 1 slow breath. The breath should last 1 to 1½ seconds.
12. Place your hand back on the compression position and give compressions. You do not have to slide your fingers up the rib cage to find the correct position.
13. Keep repeating cycles of 5 compressions and 1 breath.
14. After 10 cycles of 5 compressions and 1 breath, recheck the carotid pulse for 5 seconds. Ten cycles will take about 1 minute.
15. If there is no pulse, give 1 breath and continue CPR. Recheck the pulse every few minutes.

    If there is a pulse, check for breathing for 3 to 5 seconds. If the child is breathing, keep the airway open. Keep checking breathing and pulse closely. Look, listen, and feel for breathing. Check the pulse once every minute. Cover the child. Keep the child warm and as quiet as possible. If the child is not breathing, give rescue breathing and keep checking the pulse once every minute.
16. Continue CPR until one of the following things happens:
    - The heart starts beating again.
    - A second rescuer trained in CPR takes over for you.
    - EMS personnel arrive and take over.
    - You are too exhausted to continue.

More About CPR for a Child

If No One Comes When You Shout for Help

When you find an unconscious child, always shout for help. Shout to attract someone nearby who can phone the EMS system for help. But what if no one comes when you shout for help? You should do CPR for at least one minute. Keep shouting for help. Also plan how to make the call yourself.

If no one comes to help you after one minute of CPR, you should go to a phone as quickly as you can and call the EMS system. If possible, bring the phone where the child is or carry the child with you to the phone. Begin CPR again after you have made the call.

If a Second Trained Rescuer Is at the Scene

If another person trained in CPR is at the scene, this person should do two things: first, phone the EMS system for help if this has not been done; and second, take over CPR when you are tired. The second person should say that he or she is trained in CPR and offer to help you. If the EMS system has been called and if you are tired and ask for help, then—

1. You should stop CPR after the next breath.
2. The second rescuer should kneel next to the child across from you. Then he or she should tilt the child's head into the neutral-plus position and feel for the carotid pulse for 5 seconds.
3. If there is no pulse, the second rescuer should give 1 breath and continue CPR.
4. You should check to make sure the second rescuer is doing CPR correctly. Watch the child's chest rise and fall during rescue breathing. Feel for the carotid pulse. If you feel a pulse while compressions are being done, you know the compressions are being done correctly.

Review Questions

Check the best answer or fill in the blanks with the right word.

9. When you give CPR to a child, what is the correct cycle?
   - ☐ a. 5 compressions, then 1 breath
   - ☐ b. 10 compressions, then 2 breaths
   - ☐ c. 12 compressions, then 5 breaths

10. After you start CPR on a child, when do you check to find out if the child has a pulse?
    - ☐ a. After 2 cycles of CPR and every 4 to 5 minutes thereafter
    - ☐ b. After 10 cycles of CPR and every few minutes thereafter
    - ☐ c. Only after 20 cycles of CPR

11. When may you stop giving CPR to a child?
    - a. When the heart starts _____ again
    - b. When a second rescuer trained in _____ takes over for you
    - c. When _____ personnel arrive and take over
    - d. When you are too _____ to continue

Answers

9. a. When you give CPR to a child, the correct cycle is **5 compressions, then 1 breath.**

10. b. After starting CPR on a child, check for a pulse **after 10 cycles of CPR and every few minutes thereafter.**

11. You may stop CPR—
   a. When the heart starts **beating** again.
   b. When a second rescuer trained in **CPR** takes over for you.
   c. When **EMS** personnel arrive and take over.
   d. When you are too **exhausted** to continue.

Practice Session: CPR for a Child

During this practice session, you and a partner will practice on a manikin. **Before you start practicing,** carefully read the skill sheet on pages 105 through 114. If you don't remember how to use the skill sheet, read "Practice Sessions: Information and Directions" on pages 55 through 57.

Before you practice on the manikin, clean its face and the inside of its mouth. Directions for doing this are given in the section called "Some Health Precautions and Guidelines to Follow During This Course" on pages 3 and 4 of this workbook. **Clean the manikin's face and mouth before each person in your group practices.**

Skill Sheet: CPR for a Child

You find a child lying on the ground, not moving. You should survey the scene to see if it is safe and to get some idea of what happened. Then do a primary survey.

Partner Check
Instructor Check

☐ ☐ **Check for Unresponsiveness** (Does the child respond?)

Tap or gently shake child's shoulder.

Rescuer shouts, "Are you OK?"

Partner/Instructor says, "Unconscious."

Rescuer repeats, "Unconscious."

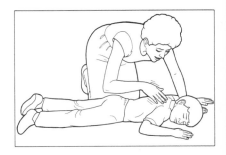

Rescuer shouts, "Help!"

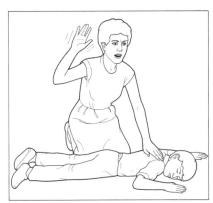

Position the Child

Place the child on his or her back.

Partner Check
Instructor Check

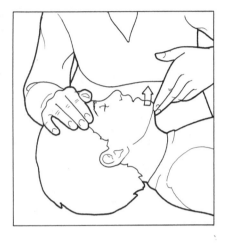

☐ ☐ **Open the Airway** (Use head-tilt/chin-lift.)

Place your hand—the one nearer the child's head—on child's forehead.

Put fingers of other hand under bony part of lower jaw at the chin.

Tilt head gently back into the neutral-plus position and lift chin. Do not close child's mouth. Do not push on the soft parts under the chin.

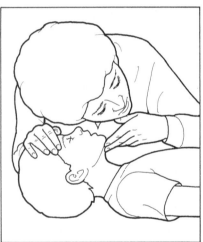

☐ ☐ **Check for Breathlessness** (Is the child breathing?)

Keep airway open with head-tilt/chin-lift.

Place your ear over child's mouth and nose.

Look at chest and abdomen. Listen and feel for breathing for 3 to 5 seconds.

Partner/Instructor says, "No breathing."

Rescuer repeats, "No breathing."

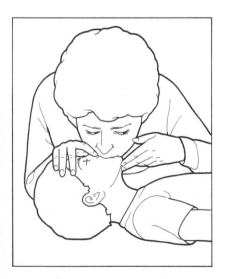

☐ ☐ **Give 2 Slow Breaths**

Keep airway open with head-tilt/chin-lift.

Pinch child's nose shut.

Open your mouth wide and take a breath. Seal your lips tightly around outside of child's mouth.

Give 2 slow breaths. Each breath should last 1 to 1½ seconds. Take a breath yourself between the breaths you give the child.

Look for the chest to rise and fall. Listen and feel for air coming out of child's nose and mouth.

Partner Check
Instructor Check

☐ ☐ **Check for Pulse**

Keep child's head tilted with one hand on forehead.

Find child's Adam's apple with middle and index fingers of your other hand.

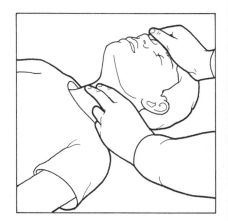

Slide fingers toward you into groove on side of neck closer to you.

Feel for carotid pulse for 5 to 10 seconds.

Partner/Instructor says, "No breathing and no pulse."

Rescuer repeats, "No breathing and no pulse."

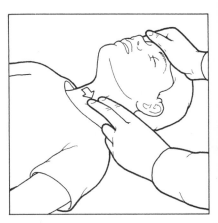

☐ ☐ **Phone the EMS System for Help**

Tell someone to call for an ambulance.

Rescuer says, "Child not breathing, has no pulse, call _____."

(Local emergency number or Operator)

Partner Check Instructor Check

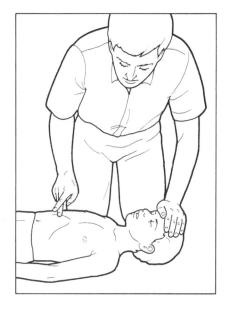

☐ ☐ **Find Compression Position**

Kneel facing child's chest.

Keep child's head tilted with hand on forehead.

With middle finger of other hand, find lower edge of child's rib cage on side closer to you.

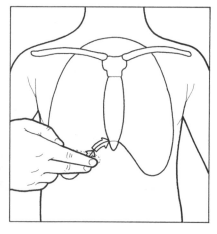

Slide middle finger up edge of rib cage to notch at lower end of breastbone.

Place middle finger in notch and index finger next to it on lower end of breastbone.

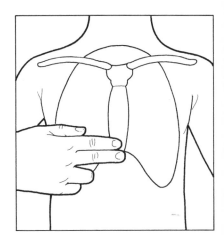

Look where your index finger is placed on child's breastbone.

Lift fingers off breastbone.

Place heel of same hand on breastbone just above where index finger was placed.

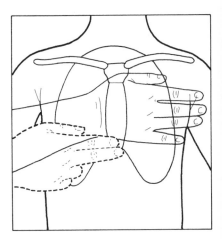

Keep fingers off child's chest.

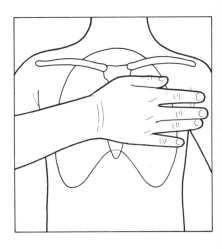

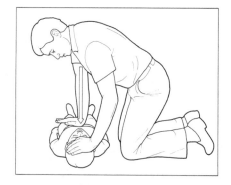

Partner Check
Instructor Check

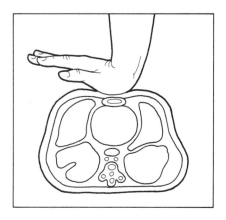

Position shoulder over hand.

☐ ☐ **Give 5 Compressions**

Compress breastbone 1 to 1½ inches (2.5 to 3.8 centimeters) at the rate of 80 to 100 compressions per minute (5 compressions should take 3 to 4 seconds).

Count out loud, "One and two and three and four and five and." (Push down as you say the number and come up as you say "and.")

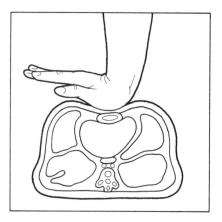

Compress down and let up smoothly, keeping your hand on the child's chest.

Keep child's head tilted with hand on forehead.

Partner Check

Instructor Check

☐ ☐ **Give 1 Slow Breath**

Keep child's head tilted with hand on forehead.

Put fingers of other hand under bony part of lower jaw at the chin. Lift chin.

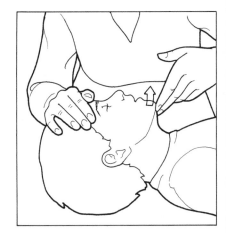

Pinch child's nose shut.

Open your mouth wide and take a breath. Seal your lips tightly around the outside of child's mouth.

Give 1 slow breath. The breath should last 1 to 1½ seconds.

Look for the chest to rise and fall. Listen and feel for air coming out of the child's nose and mouth.

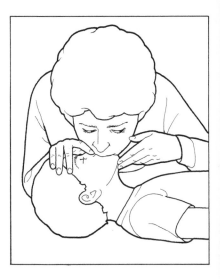

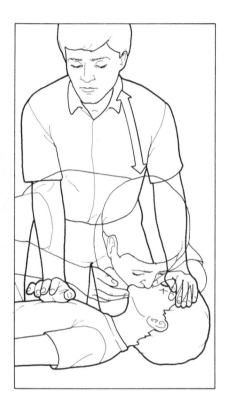

☐ ☐ **Do Compression/Breathing Cycles**

Keep child's head tilted with hand on forehead.

Put other hand back in the compression position.

Do 10 cycles of 5 compressions and 1 breath.

Partner Check
Instructor Check

☐ ☐ **Recheck Pulse**

Keep child's head tilted with hand on forehead.

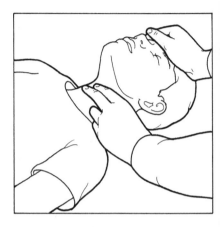

With other hand feel for carotid pulse for 5 seconds.

Partner/Instructor says, "No pulse."

Rescuer repeats, "No pulse."

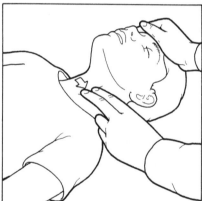

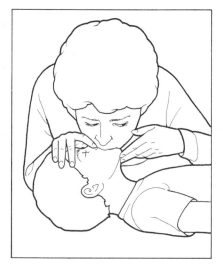

Partner Check
Instructor Check

☐ ☐ **Give 1 Slow Breath**

Keep child's head tilted with hand on forehead.

Put fingers of other hand under bony part of lower jaw at the chin. Lift chin.

Pinch child's nose shut.

Open your mouth wide and take a breath. Seal your lips tightly around outside of child's mouth.

Give 1 slow breath. The breath should last 1 to 1½ seconds.

Look for the chest to rise and fall. Listen and feel for air coming out of child's nose and mouth.

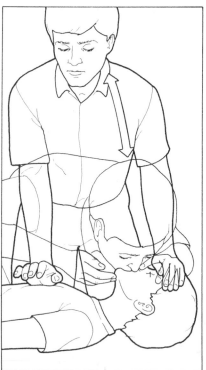

☐ ☐ **Continue Compression/Breathing Cycles**

Put hand back in compression position.

Continue cycles of 5 compressions and 1 breath.

Recheck pulse every few minutes.

☐ ☐ **What to Do Next**

When the rescuer stops to check pulse, the partner should read one of the following statements:

1. Child has a pulse.

2. Child does not have a pulse.

The rescuer should use this information to decide what to do next and then give the right care.

Final Instructor Check_____

Review Section: CPR for a Child

A three-year-old has been playing in the garage. You find her lying on the ground next to some exposed electric wires. She is not moving. You begin a primary survey. You find that she is unconscious and is not breathing. You give 2 slow breaths. Then you check the child's pulse.

1. Where should you check for a child's pulse?
- ☐ a. At the wrist
- ☐ b. On the upper arm
- ☐ c. At the side of the neck

There is no pulse. You send someone to phone for an ambulance.

2. You begin CPR. When you give CPR, what is the correct cycle?
- ☐ a. 5 compressions, then 1 breath
- ☐ b. 5 compressions, then 5 breaths
- ☐ c. 10 compressions, then 2 breaths

3. After starting CPR, when should you check for the return of a pulse?
- ☐ a. After 5 cycles of CPR and every 5 minutes thereafter
- ☐ b. After 10 cycles of CPR and every few minutes thereafter
- ☐ c. Only after 5 cycles of CPR

Answers

1. c. You should check for a child's pulse **at the side of the neck.**

2. a. When you give CPR to a child, you should do cycles of **5 compressions, then 1 breath.**

3. b. After starting CPR, you should check for the return of a pulse **after 10 cycles of CPR and every few minutes thereafter.**

6

What to Do When an Infant's Breathing Stops (Rescue Breathing)

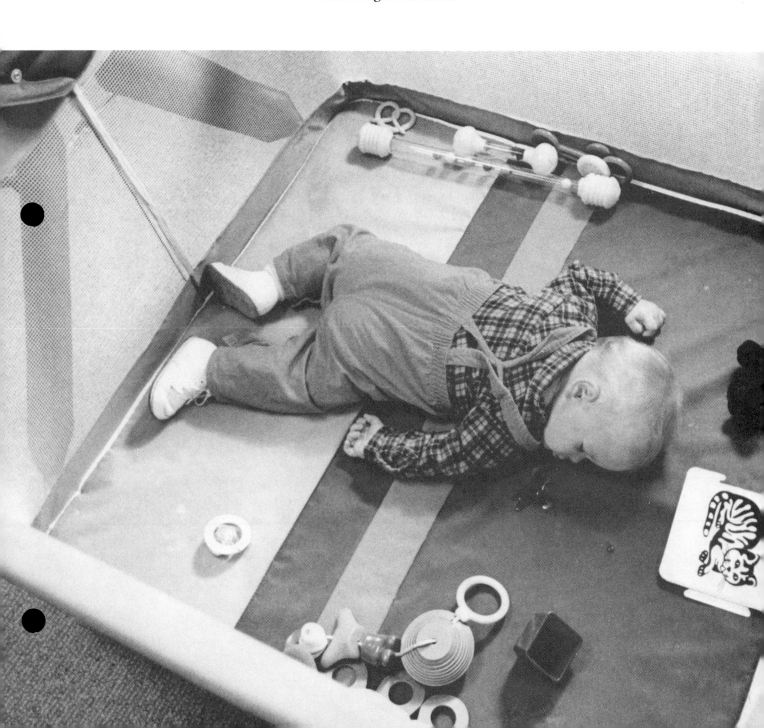

In Chapter 3, you learned how to give rescue breathing to a child. In this chapter, you will learn how to give rescue breathing to an infant younger than one year old.

Objectives

By the time you finish reading this chapter, you should be able to do the following:

1. Describe the early signals of a breathing emergency.
2. Describe when an infant needs rescue breathing.
3. Describe how to position an infant for rescue breathing.
4. Describe how to give rescue breathing to an infant.

Breathing Emergencies in Infants

When an infant stops breathing, this is a breathing emergency. Breathing emergencies happen in different ways. A breathing emergency can happen when an infant is injured in a motor vehicle accident or suffers burns or breathes smoke. Poisoning, suffocation, and near-drowning can cause an infant to stop breathing. An infant will also stop breathing if the airway becomes blocked. Sometimes a medical condition or an illness, such as severe croup, causes a breathing emergency.

It is important to recognize the early signals of a breathing emergency. These signals warn you that a breathing emergency is about to happen. Look for any of these signals:

- Infant is agitated or excited.
- Infant seems drowsy.
- Infant's skin color changes (to pale, blue, or gray).
- Infant is having difficulty breathing.
- Infant is breathing faster.
- Infant's heart is beating faster.

If you believe an infant is having a breathing emergency, you should give first aid. The first aid for an infant whose breathing has stopped but whose heart is beating is called rescue breathing.

How to Give Rescue Breathing to an Infant

If you find an infant lying very still and suspect that something might be wrong, you should quickly survey the scene and do a primary survey.

1. **Check for Unresponsiveness**

    The first thing you should do is check to see if the infant is conscious. Tap or gently shake the infant's shoulder to see if he or she responds *(Fig. 38)*. Does the infant move or make a noise?

2. **Shout for Help**

    If the infant does not move or make a noise, shout for help *(Fig. 39)*. You do this to get the attention of people you can ask to phone the EMS system for help after you do a primary survey.

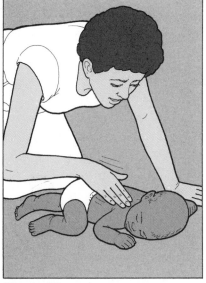

Figure 38
Check for Unresponsiveness

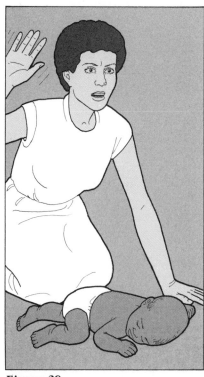

Figure 39
Shout for Help

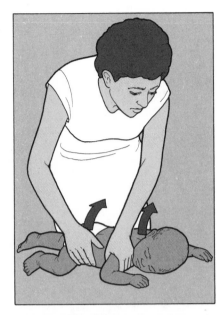

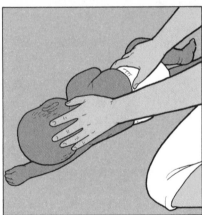

Figure 40
Position the Infant

3. Position the Infant

Move the infant onto his or her back. To do this, roll the infant as a unit *(Fig. 40).* This will help to avoid twisting the body and making any injuries worse. To position the infant—

- Stand or kneel facing the infant.
- Straighten the infant's legs, if necessary.
- Move the infant's arm—the one closer to you—so that it is stretched out above the infant's head.
- Lean over the infant and place one hand on the infant's shoulder. Put your other hand on the infant's hip.
- Roll the infant toward you as a unit by pulling slowly and evenly. Don't let the infant's head and body twist.
- Move your hand from the shoulder to support the back of the head and neck as you roll the infant.
- Place the infant's arm—the one closer to you—beside the infant's body.

It is important to position the infant on his or her back as quickly as possible.

Note: Some infants who require rescue breathing or CPR may have received a serious injury to the head, neck, or back. Moving these infants, or opening the airway as described below, could result in further injury. If you think the infant might have a serious head, neck, or back injury, don't move the infant. Additional methods for handling these infants are discussed in the American Red Cross CPR: Basic Life Support for the Professional Rescuer course.

4. **"A"—Open the Airway**

   Open the infant's airway using the head-tilt/chin-lift *(Fig. 41)*. This is the most important step you can take to help the infant live. To open the airway—

   - Stand or kneel beside the infant's head.
   - Put your hand—the one nearer the infant's head—on the infant's forehead.
   - Put one finger (not the thumb) of your other hand under the bony part of the infant's lower jaw at the chin.
   - Tilt the infant's head gently back into the neutral position by applying pressure on the forehead and lifting the chin. The neutral position is shown in *Figure 42*. Do not close the infant's mouth completely. Do not push in on the soft parts under the chin.

5. **"B"—Check for Breathlessness** (Look, listen, and feel for breathing.)

   With the infant's head in the neutral position and the chin lifted, check to see if the infant is breathing *(Fig. 43)*. Tilting the head into the neutral position and lifting the chin opens the airway. This may help the infant start breathing again. To check the infant's breathing—

   - Place your ear just over the infant's mouth and nose. Look at the infant's chest and abdomen.
   - Look, listen, and feel. **Look** for the chest and abdomen to rise and fall. **Listen** for breathing. **Feel** for air coming out of the infant's nose and mouth against your ear and cheek. Do this for 3 to 5 seconds.

   If the infant is breathing, you will see the chest and abdomen move. You will hear and feel air coming out of the infant's nose and mouth. Movement of the chest and abdomen does not always mean that the infant is breathing. The infant may be trying unsuccessfully to breathe. Be sure to look, listen, and feel for breathing.

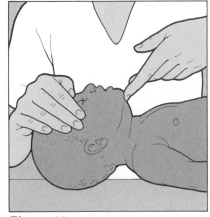

Figure 41
Head-Tilt/Chin-Lift

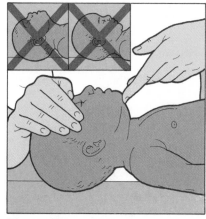

Figure 42
Tilt Head Into Neutral Position and Lift Chin

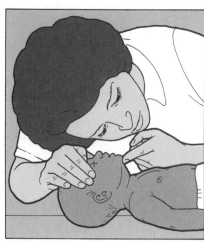

Figure 43
Check for Breathlessness

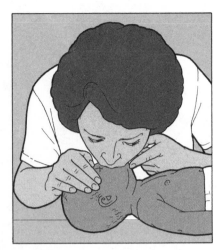

Figure 44
Mouth-to-Mouth-and-Nose Breathing

6. **Give 2 Slow Breaths**

   If the infant is not breathing, you must get air into the lungs at once *(Fig. 44)*. To give breaths—
   - Keep the airway open with the head-tilt/chin-lift. Open your mouth wide and take a breath. Seal your lips tightly around the infant's mouth and nose.
   - Give 2 slow breaths. Each breath should last 1 to 1½ seconds. Remove your mouth between breaths just long enough for you to take a breath. Watch for the chest to rise while you breathe into the infant. Watch for the chest to fall after each breath. Listen and feel for air coming out of the nose and mouth.

   If air will not go into the infant's lungs easily, retilt the head and give 2 more breaths. If air still does not go into the infant's lungs, the airway may be blocked by food or some other material. Chapter 7 describes how to help an infant with a blocked airway.

   Because an infant's airway is smaller than an adult's, it may be difficult to breathe air into the lungs. Be careful not to breathe too hard. If you blow too fast and too forcefully into the infant's airway, you can cause air to go into the stomach. On the other hand, if you blow too softly, you will not fill the infant's lungs with air. You should breathe slowly and watch for the chest to rise. When the chest rises, stop breathing into the infant.

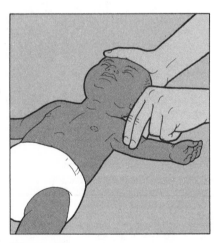

Figure 45
Locate Brachial Pulse

7. **"C"—Check Circulation by Checking for a Pulse in the Upper Arm**

   Check to see if the infant's heart is beating by feeling for a pulse in the upper arm closer to you. This pulse is called the **brachial pulse** *(Fig. 45)*. It is located on the inside of the upper arm between the elbow and the shoulder. To check for a brachial pulse—
   - Keep one hand on the infant's forehead to keep the head in the neutral position.
   - Use your other hand to find the pulse in the infant's arm closer to you. Press gently with your index and middle fingers on the inside of the arm between the elbow and the shoulder.
   - Feel for the brachial pulse with your fingers for 5 to 10 seconds.

8. **Phone the EMS System**

   After you have checked the pulse, you will have the information the EMS dispatcher needs. Before you send the bystanders to phone, tell them whether the infant is conscious, breathing, and has a pulse. Tell them to give this information to the EMS dispatcher.

9. Begin Rescue Breathing

If you feel a pulse and the infant is not breathing, then begin rescue breathing. (If you do not feel a pulse, the infant's heart has stopped. You must start CPR, which you will learn in Chapter 8.) To give rescue breathing—

- Keep the infant's airway open using the head-tilt/chin-lift.
- Open your mouth wide and take a breath. Seal your lips tightly around the outside of the infant's mouth and nose. Give 1 breath every 3 seconds. Each breath should last for 1 to 1½ seconds. A good way to time the breaths is to count, "One one-thousand, two one-thousand." Take a breath yourself and then breathe into the infant. Watch for the chest to rise as you breathe into the infant.
- Between breaths, remove your mouth from the infant. Look for the chest to fall as you listen and feel at the infant's mouth and nose for air to come out. Listen to hear if the infant starts breathing again.

10. Recheck Pulse

After 1 minute of rescue breathing (about 20 breaths), you should check the infant's pulse. To check the pulse—

- Keep the infant's head in the neutral position with one hand on the infant's forehead.
- With the other hand, feel for the brachial pulse for 5 seconds.

If the infant has a pulse, then check for breathing for 3 to 5 seconds.

If the infant is breathing, keep the airway open. Keep checking breathing and pulse closely. Look, listen, and feel for breathing. Check the pulse once every minute. Cover the infant. Keep the infant warm and as quiet as possible.

If the infant is not breathing, continue rescue breathing. Check the pulse once every minute. Continue giving rescue breathing until—

- The infant begins breathing on his or her own.
- Another trained rescuer takes over for you.
- EMS personnel arrive and take over.
- You are too exhausted to continue.

Review Questions

Check the best answer or fill in the blanks with the right word.

1. You find an infant lying very still on the floor. You think something is wrong. You survey the scene and decide it is safe. What should you do when you reach the infant?
    ☐ a. Check for unresponsiveness.
    ☐ b. Check the infant's pulse.
    ☐ c. Begin rescue breathing.

2. When should you give rescue breathing to an infant?
    ☐ a. When the infant is breathing and has a pulse
    ☐ b. When the infant's heart has stopped beating
    ☐ c. When the infant is not breathing but has a pulse

3. Where should you place your finger when doing the chin-lift on an infant?
    ☐ a. Under the bony part of the lower jaw at the chin
    ☐ b. On the Adam's apple
    ☐ c. Under the back of the infant's neck

4. Where should you check for an infant's brachial pulse?

☐ a. In the groove between the windpipe and the muscle at the side of the neck

☐ b. On the inside of the wrist

☐ c. On the inside of the upper arm between the elbow and the shoulder

5. How often should you give rescue breaths to an infant?

☐ a. Give 1 breath every second.

☐ b. Give 1 breath every 3 seconds.

☐ c. Give 1 breath every 10 seconds.

6. You should continue rescue breathing until one of four things happens. These four things are—

a. The infant starts _____.

b. Another _____ rescuer takes over for you.

c. _____ personnel arrive and take over.

d. You are too _____ to continue.

Answers

1. **a.** If you find an infant lying very still and you think something is wrong, the first thing you should do is **check for unresponsiveness.**

2. **c.** You should give rescue breathing **when the infant is not breathing but has a pulse.**

3. **a.** When doing the chin-lift on an infant, you should place your finger **under the bony part of the lower jaw at the chin.**

4. **c.** You should check for an infant's brachial pulse **on the inside of the upper arm between the elbow and the shoulder.**

5. **b.** For an infant, **give 1 breath every 3 seconds.**

6. You should continue rescue breathing until one of the following happens:
   a. The infant starts **breathing.**
   b. Another **trained** rescuer takes over for you.
   c. **EMS** personnel arrive and take over.
   d. You are too **exhausted** to continue.

More About Rescue Breathing for an Infant

Air in the Stomach

Sometimes while doing rescue breathing, you may breathe air into the infant's stomach. Air in the stomach can be a serious problem because it makes the stomach swell. Then the lungs do not have enough room to fill with air when you give rescue breaths. Therefore, the infant may not get enough oxygen to live.

To keep from forcing air into the infant's stomach, do the following:

- **Keep the infant's head in the neutral position** to keep the airway open. If you feel that the air is not going in easily, tilt the infant's head back a little farther and continue rescue breathing.
- **Give slow breaths.** Each breath should last 1 to 1½ seconds.
- **Breathe only enough air to make the chest rise.** Let the chest fall before you give the infant another breath.

Vomiting

Sometimes while you are helping an unconscious infant, he or she may vomit. It is important that the vomit does not get into the lungs. If the infant vomits, quickly turn the infant's head and body to the side. Wipe out the infant's mouth and continue rescue breathing.

Practice Session: Rescue Breathing for an Infant

During this practice session, you and a partner will practice on a manikin. You will practice the steps and will give actual rescue breaths. **Before you start practicing,** carefully read the skill sheet on pages 128 through 132. If you don't remember how to use the skill sheet, read "Practice Sessions: Information and Directions" on pages 55 through 57.

Before you practice on the manikin, clean its face and the inside of its mouth. Directions for doing this are given in the section called "Some Health Precautions and Guidelines to Follow During This Course" on pages 3 and 4 of this workbook. **Clean the manikin's face and mouth before each person in your group practices.**

Skill Sheet: Rescue Breathing for an Infant

You find an infant lying unusually still, and you suspect that something may be wrong. You should survey the scene to see if it is safe and to get some idea of what happened. Then do a primary survey.

□ □ **Check for Unresponsiveness** (Does the infant respond?)

Tap or gently shake infant's shoulder.

Partner/Instructor says, "Unconscious."

Rescuer repeats, "Unconscious."

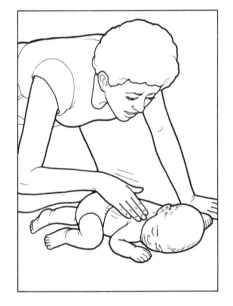

Rescuer shouts, "Help!"

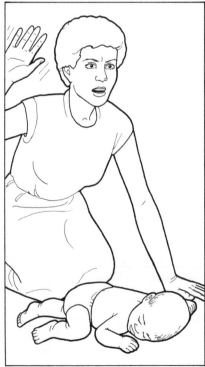

Position the Infant

Roll infant onto back, if necessary.

Stand or kneel facing infant.

Straighten infant's legs, if necessary, and move infant's arm—the one closer to you—above infant's head.

Lean over infant and place one hand on infant's shoulder and your other hand on infant's hip.

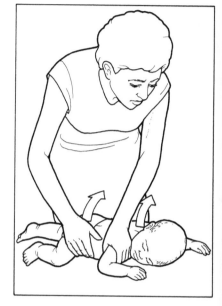

Roll infant toward you as a unit. As you roll infant, move your hand from infant's shoulder to support back of head and neck.

Place infant's arm—the one closer to you—beside infant's body.

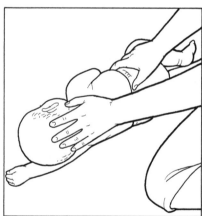

Partner Check
Instructor Check

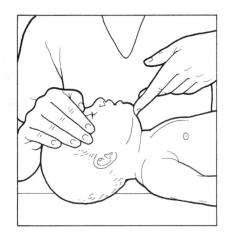

☐ ☐ **Open the Airway** (Use head-tilt/chin-lift.)

Put your hand—the one nearer the infant's head—on infant's forehead.

Put finger of other hand under bony part of lower jaw at the chin.

Tilt head gently back into the neutral position and lift chin. Do not close infant's mouth completely. Do not push on the soft parts under the chin.

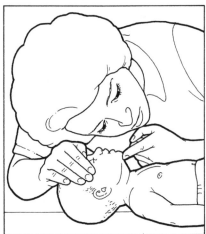

☐ ☐ **Check for Breathlessness** (Is the infant breathing?)

Keep airway open with head-tilt/chin-lift.

Place your ear over infant's mouth and nose.

Look at chest and abdomen. Listen and feel for breathing for 3 to 5 seconds.

Partner/Instructor says, "No breathing."

Rescuer repeats, "No breathing."

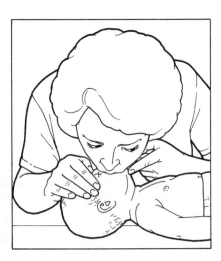

☐ ☐ **Give 2 Slow Breaths**

Keep airway open with head-tilt/chin-lift.

Open your mouth wide and take a breath. Seal your lips tightly around infant's mouth and nose.

Give 2 slow breaths. Each breath should last 1 to 1½ seconds. Take a breath yourself between the breaths you give the infant.

Look for the chest to rise and fall. Listen and feel for air coming out of the infant's nose and mouth.

Partner Check
Instructor Check

☐ ☐ **Check for Pulse**

Keep infant's head tilted with one hand on forehead.

With other hand press gently with your index and middle fingers on inside of upper arm.

Feel for brachial pulse for 5 to 10 seconds.

Partner/Instructor says, "No breathing, but there is a pulse."

Rescuer repeats, "No breathing, but there is a pulse."

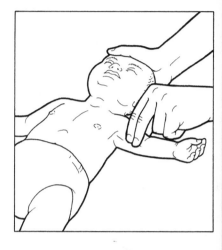

☐ ☐ **Phone the EMS System for Help**

Tell someone to call for an ambulance.

Rescuer says, "Infant not breathing, but has a pulse, call _____."
(Local emergency number or Operator)

☐ ☐ **Now Begin Rescue Breathing**

Keep airway open with head-tilt/chin-lift.

Open your mouth wide and take a breath. Seal your lips tightly around infant's mouth and nose.

Give 1 breath every 3 seconds. Each breath should last 1 to 1½ seconds. Count aloud, "One one-thousand, two one-thousand." Take a breath yourself and then breathe into the infant.

Look for the chest to rise and fall. Listen and feel for air coming out of the infant's nose and mouth.

Do rescue breathing for 1 minute—about 20 breaths.

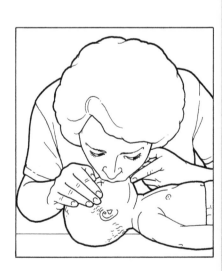

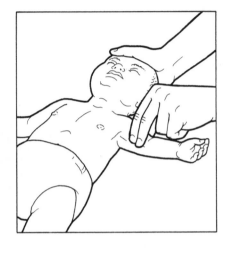

Partner Check

Instructor Check

□ □ **Recheck Pulse**

Keep infant's head tilted with one hand on forehead.

With other hand feel for brachial pulse for 5 seconds.

Partner/Instructor says, "Has a pulse."

Rescuer repeats, "Has a pulse."

Look, listen, and feel for breathing for 3 to 5 seconds.

Partner/Instructor says, "No breathing."

Rescuer repeats, "No breathing."

□ □ **Continue Rescue Breathing**

Keep airway open with head-tilt/chin-lift.

Give 1 breath every 3 seconds. Each breath should last 1 to 1½ seconds.

Recheck pulse once every minute.

□ □ **What to Do Next**

While the rescuer is rechecking pulse and breathing, the partner should read one of the following statements:

1. Infant is breathing but is still unconscious.

2. Infant has a pulse but is not breathing.

The rescuer should use this information to decide what to do next and then give the right care.

Final Instructor Check_____

Review Section: Rescue Breathing for an Infant

You hear your neighbor shouting, "Help!" She says she found her infant lying in the crib with a big stuffed toy over her face. You check for unresponsiveness. The infant is unconscious. You check the ABCs.

1. Fill in the blanks in the following statements:

   A—Airway   You open the airway by doing the head-tilt/ _____ -lift. The infant's head should be tilted into the neutral position.

   B—Breathing   When you check for breathing, you look, _____, and feel for breathing.

   C—Circulation   You check the infant's pulse by pressing gently against the inside of the upper _____.

   The infant is not breathing but has a pulse. You tell your neighbor to phone the EMS system for help.

2. What should you do next?
   - [ ] a. Check the infant's pulse.
   - [ ] b. Begin rescue breathing.
   - [ ] c. Check for breathing again.

3. How often should you recheck the infant's pulse?
   - [ ] a. After 1 minute and once every minute thereafter
   - [ ] b. After 2 minutes and every 5 minutes thereafter
   - [ ] c. After 4 minutes and every 5 minutes thereafter

   You find that there is a pulse but the infant is still not breathing. You continue rescue breathing.

4. How often should you give rescue breaths to an infant?
   - [ ] a. Give 1 breath every second.
   - [ ] b. Give 1 breath every 3 seconds.
   - [ ] c. Give 1 breath every 6 seconds.

Answers

1. You open the airway by doing the head-tilt/**chin**-lift.

   When you check for breathing, you look, **listen,** and feel for breathing.

   You check an infant's pulse by pressing gently against the inside of the upper **arm.**

2. **b.** When an infant is not breathing but has a pulse, you should **begin rescue breathing.**

3. **a.** You should recheck the infant's pulse **after 1 minute and once every minute thereafter.**

4. **b.** For an infant, you should **give 1 breath every 3 seconds.**

7

What to Do for an Infant Who Is Choking

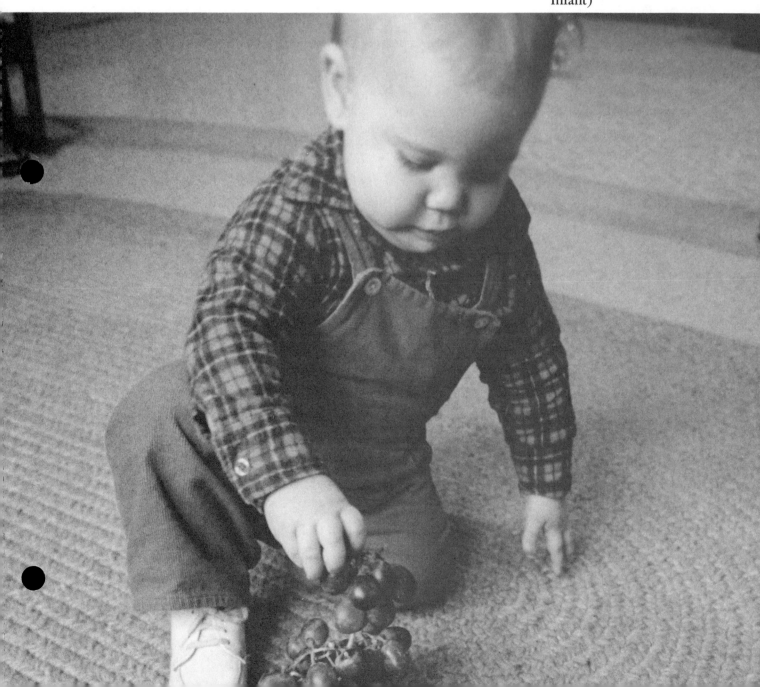

In Chapter 4, you learned first aid for a child who is choking. In this chapter, you will learn what to do when an infant is choking. When this happens, the infant can quickly stop breathing, lose consciousness, and die. You will learn how to tell if a choking infant needs first aid. You will also learn the first aid to clear a blocked airway.

Objectives

By the time you finish reading this chapter, you should be able to do the following:

1. *Describe the signals of choking in a conscious infant.*
2. *Describe the first aid for a conscious infant who is choking.*
3. *Describe how you would find out that an unconscious infant has a blocked airway.*
4. *Describe the first aid for an unconscious infant with a blocked airway.*
5. *Describe the first aid for a conscious infant who becomes unconscious while choking.*

Causes and Signals of Choking

Choking is a major cause of death and injury in infants. One reason is that infants find out about their world by putting objects in their mouth. Small objects such as pebbles, coins, beads, and parts of toys are dangerous if an infant swallows them. Infants also often choke because it takes a long time to develop their eating skills. First they suck from a bottle or breast. Then they are fed soft foods. Finally, they learn to feed themselves. As they grow teeth, they can eat more and more kinds of food. But infants can easily choke on some foods that an adult can eat, such as nuts, grapes, or popcorn.

To prevent choking, never let an infant eat alone. Never prop up a bottle for an infant to drink alone. Always stay with an infant during meals or snacks. Cut food into small pieces. Do not give an infant foods such as nuts that could lodge in the airway. If you suspect that an infant has an object in his or her mouth, check with your fingers and remove it. Regularly check floors, rugs, and other places for pins, coins, and other small objects that an infant might pick up and put in his or her mouth.

A choking infant can quickly stop breathing, lose consciousness, and die. Therefore, it is very important to recognize when an infant needs first aid for choking. These are signals that an infant is choking:

- **The infant coughs forcefully.** This can be a signal that the infant's airway is partially blocked but that the infant is still able to breathe.

 If an infant is coughing forcefully, stay with the infant. Watch the infant carefully. If the infant does not stop coughing soon, call the EMS system for help.

- **The infant coughs weakly or makes a high-pitched sound** while breathing. These signals mean that an infant's airway is partially blocked and that the infant cannot breathe properly. You should give first aid to clear the airway.

- **The infant cannot cry, cough, or breathe.** This means that the infant's airway is completely blocked. You should give first aid to clear the airway.

Review Questions

Check the best answer.

1. An infant is choking on some food. She is conscious and is coughing forcefully. What should you do?
   - ☐ a. Do abdominal thrusts.
   - ☐ b. Watch the infant carefully.
   - ☐ c. Pat the infant gently on the back.

2. A conscious infant is choking and is coughing weakly. What should you do?
   - ☐ a. Give first aid to clear the airway.
   - ☐ b. Watch the infant carefully.
   - ☐ c. Do abdominal thrusts.

Answers

1. **b.** If a choking infant is conscious and is coughing forcefully, you should **watch the infant carefully.**

2. **a.** You should **give first aid to clear the airway** if a conscious infant is choking and is coughing weakly.

First Aid for Choking (Conscious Infant)

You should give first aid for a blocked airway if—
- The infant cannot cough, breathe, or cry.
- The choking infant is coughing weakly or making a high-pitched sound.

If you suspect that an infant is choking, you should survey the scene as you approach the infant.

1. Begin a primary survey. Determine if the infant can cough, breathe, or cry.
2. If you are alone, shout for help.
3. Have someone phone the EMS system for help.
4. Give 4 back blows as follows:
   - Hold the infant's jaw between your thumb and fingers *(Fig. 46).*
   - Slide your other hand behind the infant's back so that your fingers support the back of the infant's head and neck.
   - Turn the infant over so that he or she is facedown on your forearm *(Fig. 47).*
   - Support the infant's head and neck with your hand by firmly holding the jaw between your thumb and fingers.

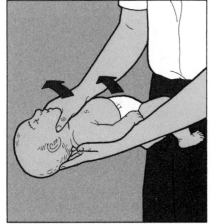

Figure 46
Hold Infant's Jaw

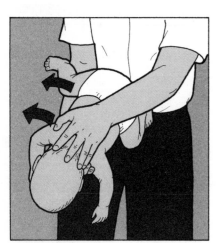

Figure 47
Turn Infant Over

- Lower your arm onto your thigh. The infant's head should be lower than his or her chest.
- Give 4 back blows forcefully between the infant's shoulder blades with the heel of your hand *(Fig. 48)*.

5. Then give 4 chest thrusts as follows:
- Place your free hand and forearm along the infant's head and back so that the infant is sandwiched between your two hands and forearms.
- Support the back of the infant's head and neck with your fingers *(Fig. 49)*.
- Support the infant's neck, jaw, and chest from the front with one hand while you support the infant's back with your other hand and forearm.

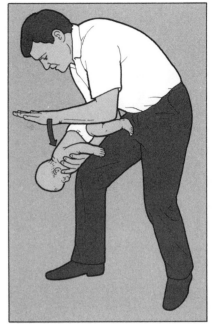

Figure 48
Give 4 Back Blows

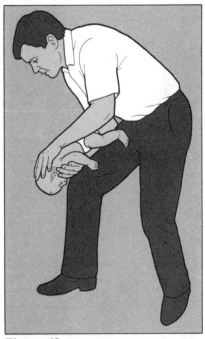

Figure 49
Support Back of Infant's Head and Neck

- Turn the infant onto his or her back *(Fig. 50)*.
- Lower your arm that is supporting the infant's back onto your thigh. The infant's head should be lower than his or her chest. (If the infant is large or your hands are too small to support the infant, put the infant on your lap with his or her head lower than the chest.)
- Use your hand that is on the infant's chest to locate the correct place to give chest thrusts. Imagine a line running across the infant's chest between the nipples *(Fig. 51)*. Place the pad of your ring finger on the breastbone just under this imaginary line *(Fig. 52)*. Then place the pads of two fingers next to your ring finger just under the nipple line. Raise your ring finger. If you feel the notch at the end of the infant's breastbone, move your fingers slightly toward the head. The pads of your fingers should lie in the same direction as the infant's breastbone.
- Use these two fingers to compress the breastbone *(Fig. 53)*. Compress the breastbone ½ to 1 inch (1.3 to 2.5 centimeters), and then let the breastbone return to its normal position. Keep your fingers in contact with the infant's breastbone. Compress 4 times.

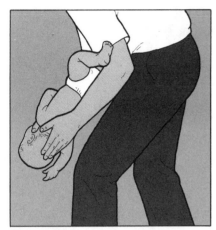

Figure 50
Turn Infant Onto Back

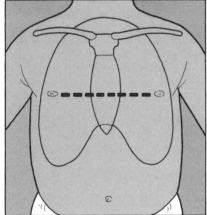

Figure 51
Imaginary Line Between Nipples

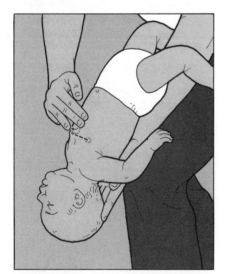

Figure 52
Locate Position for Chest Thrusts

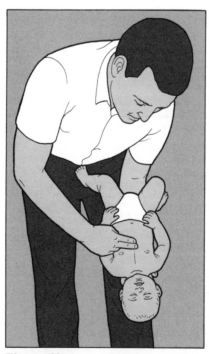

Figure 53
Position for Giving Chest Thrusts

6. Keep giving the infant back blows and chest thrusts until the object is coughed up or the infant loses consciousness.

Later in this chapter, you will learn how to help a choking infant who becomes unconscious.

When to Stop

Stop giving back blows and chest thrusts if the object is coughed up or the infant starts to breathe or cough. Watch the infant, and make sure that the infant is breathing freely again. Even after the infant coughs up the object, he or she may have breathing and lung problems that will need a doctor's attention. You should also realize that chest thrusts may cause internal injuries. For these reasons, you should call the EMS system if you have not already done so. **The infant should be taken to the hospital emergency department to be checked by a doctor. Do this even if he or she seems to be breathing well.**

Review Questions

Check the best answer.

3. When you are giving back blows and chest thrusts to a choking infant, where should the infant's head be?
- ☐ a. Lower than the chest
- ☐ b. On the same level as the chest
- ☐ c. Higher than the chest

4. When you give back blows to a choking infant, where should you place your hand?
- ☐ a. On the back of the neck
- ☐ b. Between the shoulder blades
- ☐ c. In the middle of the back at waist level

5. When you give back blows, what part of your hand should you use?
- ☐ a. The palm
- ☐ b. The heel
- ☐ c. The knuckles

6. When you give chest thrusts to an infant, where should you place your fingers?
- ☐ a. On the breastbone, just below the nipples
- ☐ b. Just above the navel and well below the lower tip of the breastbone
- ☐ c. On the navel

Answers

3. a. When you are giving back blows and chest thrusts to an infant, the infant's head should be **lower than the chest.**

4. b. When you give back blows to an infant, you should place your hand **between the shoulder blades.**

5. b. When you give back blows, you should use **the heel** of your hand.

6. a. When you give chest thrusts to an infant, you should place your fingers **on the breastbone, just below the nipples.**

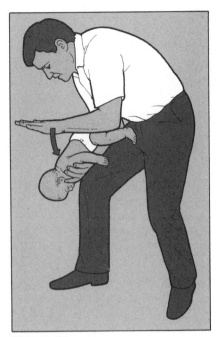

Figure 54
Give 4 Back Blows

First Aid for Choking (Unconscious Infant)

First aid for any unconscious infant begins with a primary survey. While checking the ABCs, you may find that an infant has a blocked airway. The procedure for finding out if an unconscious infant has a blocked airway is given below. First, survey the scene. Then do a primary survey.

1. Check for unresponsiveness.
2. Shout for help.
3. Position the infant on his or her back on a firm, flat surface.
4. Open the airway.
5. Look, listen, and feel for breathing for 3 to 5 seconds.
6. Give 2 slow breaths.
7. If you are unable to breathe air into the infant, retilt the head and give 2 more breaths. You may not have tilted the infant's head into the correct position the first time.

If you still cannot breathe air into the infant, tell someone to phone the EMS system for help, and do the following:

8. Give 4 back blows *(Fig. 54)* (as explained on pages 138 and 139).
9. Give 4 chest thrusts *(Fig. 55)* (as explained on pages 139 and 140).
10. Do a foreign-body check (as explained on page 143).
11. Open the airway and give 2 slow breaths.

Repeat steps 8, 9, 10, and 11 until the airway is clear or EMS personnel arrive and take over.

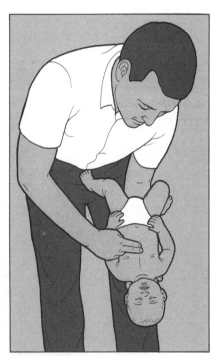

Figure 55
Give 4 Chest Thrusts

Foreign-Body Check

To do a foreign-body check—

- Stand or kneel beside the infant's head.
- Open the infant's mouth using your hand that is nearer the infant's feet. Put your thumb into the infant's mouth and hold both the tongue and the lower jaw between your thumb and fingers *(Fig. 56)*. Lift the jaw upward. This will bring the tongue away from the back of the throat and away from any object that may be lodged there.
- Look for the object, and, only if you can see it, try to remove it by doing a finger sweep.

To do the finger sweep—

- Slide the little finger of your other hand into the infant's mouth. Slide your finger down along the inside of the cheek to the base of the tongue *(Fig. 57)*. Be careful not to push the object deeper into the airway.
- Use a hooking action to loosen the object and move it into the mouth so that it can be removed. If you can reach the object, take it out.

Remember: Do the finger sweep only if you can see the object in the infant's throat.

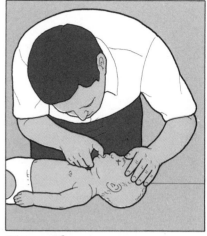

Figure 56
Foreign-Body Check

2 Slow Breaths

After you do the foreign-body check, give 2 slow breaths as follows:

- Open the airway with the head-tilt/chin-lift.
- Give 2 slow breaths.

Continue these four steps:

1. Give 4 back blows.
2. Give 4 chest thrusts.
3. Do a foreign-body check.
4. Open the airway and give 2 slow breaths.

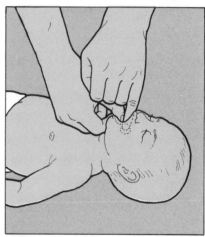

Figure 57
Finger Sweep for an Infant

If your first attempts to clear the airway are unsuccessful, do not stop. The longer the infant goes without oxygen, the more the muscles of the throat will relax. This will make it more likely that you will be able to remove the object.

If you are able to breathe air into the infant's lungs, give 2 slow breaths as you did for rescue breathing. Then check the infant's pulse. If there is no pulse, begin CPR, which you will learn in Chapter 8. If there is a pulse and the infant is not breathing on his or her own, continue rescue breathing.

If the infant starts breathing on his or her own, keep checking breathing and pulse until EMS personnel arrive and take over. This means you should keep the airway open. Look, listen, and feel for breathing. Keep checking the pulse. Cover the infant. Keep the infant warm and as quiet as possible.

Put the Steps Together

These are the steps for helping an unconscious infant whose airway may be blocked:

1. Check for unresponsiveness.
2. Shout for help.
3. Position the infant on his or her back on a firm, flat surface.
4. Open the airway.
5. Look, listen, and feel for breathing for 3 to 5 seconds.
6. If the infant is not breathing, give 2 slow breaths.
7. Retilt the head if you cannot breathe air into the infant.
8. Give 2 slow breaths.

If you are able to breathe air into the infant's lungs, give 2 slow breaths as you did for rescue breathing. Then check the infant's pulse. If there is no pulse, begin CPR, which you will learn in Chapter 8. If there is a pulse, check for breathing. If the infant is not breathing on his or her own, continue rescue breathing.

9. Give 4 back blows.
10. Give 4 chest thrusts.
11. Do a foreign-body check.
12. Open the airway and give 2 slow breaths.

Repeat steps 9, 10, 11, and 12 in the same order until the airway is clear or EMS personnel arrive and take over. If you succeed in removing the object, open the airway and give 2 slow breaths. Then check for a pulse. If there is no pulse, begin CPR. If there is a pulse, check for breathing. If the infant is not breathing on his or her own, continue rescue breathing.

Review Questions

Check the best answer.

7. An unconscious infant is not breathing. If you cannot breathe air into the infant's lungs on the first try, what should you do next?
   - ☐ a. Retilt the head and give 2 slow breaths.
   - ☐ b. Do a foreign-body check.
   - ☐ c. Give back blows and chest thrusts.

8. An unconscious infant has a blocked airway. How many back blows and chest thrusts should you give before you do a foreign-body check?
   - ☐ a. 4 back blows and 2 chest thrusts.
   - ☐ b. 6 back blows and 4 chest thrusts.
   - ☐ c. 4 back blows and 4 chest thrusts.

9. You remove an object from an infant's mouth with a finger sweep. You give 2 slow breaths and see the infant's chest rise and fall. What should you do next?
   - ☐ a. Open the airway.
   - ☐ b. Check the pulse.
   - ☐ c. Phone the EMS system for help.

10. When should you do a finger sweep on an infant?
   - ☐ a. Only when you can see an object in the infant's throat
   - ☐ b. When the second set of 2 slow breaths will not go into the infant's lungs
   - ☐ c. When you think the infant has swallowed an object

Answers

7. **a.** **Retilt the head and give 2 slow breaths** if you cannot breathe air into an unconscious infant who is not breathing.

8. **c.** You should give **4 back blows and 4 chest thrusts** to an unconscious infant before doing a foreign-body check.

9. **b.** If you are able to breathe air into the infant, the next thing you should do is **check the pulse.**

10. **a.** You should do a finger sweep on an infant **only when you can see an object in the infant's throat.**

First Aid for Choking When a Conscious Infant Becomes Unconscious

If an infant becomes unconscious while you are giving first aid for choking, you should shout for help. Have someone phone the EMS system for help if it hasn't already been done. Place the infant on a firm, flat surface. Then—

1. Do a foreign-body check.
2. Open the airway and give 2 slow breaths.
3. Give 4 back blows.
4. Give 4 chest thrusts.

Repeat these four steps until the airway is clear or EMS personnel arrive and take over.

If you are able to breathe air into the infant's lungs, give 2 slow breaths as you did for rescue breathing. Then check the pulse. If the infant has no pulse, then you must begin CPR. If there is a pulse and the infant is not breathing on his or her own, continue rescue breathing.

If the infant starts breathing on his or her own, keep checking breathing and pulse until EMS personnel arrive and take over. This means you should keep the airway open. Look, listen, and feel for breathing. Keep checking the pulse. Cover the infant. Keep the infant warm and as quiet as possible.

Practice Sessions: First Aid for Choking

First, you will learn first aid for a conscious infant with a blocked airway. Later on, you will learn first aid for an unconscious infant with a blocked airway.

Practice Session 1: First Aid for Choking (Conscious Infant)
You will learn the first aid for a conscious infant with a blocked airway. You will practice this skill on a manikin.

    Before you start practicing, carefully read the skill sheet on pages 148 through 152. If you don't remember how to use the skill sheet, read "Practice Sessions: Information and Directions" on pages 55 through 57. When you practice, do not touch the manikin's lips or inside the mouth with your fingers.

Practice Session 2: First Aid for Choking (Unconscious Infant)
You will learn the first aid for an unconscious infant with a blocked airway. You will practice this skill on a manikin.

    Before you start practicing, carefully read the skill sheet on pages 153 through 160. If you don't remember how to use the skill sheet, read "Practice Sessions: Information and Directions" on pages 55 through 57.

    When you practice, do not touch the manikin's lips or inside the mouth with your fingers. Before you practice on the manikin, clean its face and the inside of its mouth. Directions for doing this are given in the section called "Some Health Precautions and Guidelines to Follow During This Course" on pages 3 and 4 of this workbook. **Clean the manikin's face and mouth before each person in your group practices.**

Skill Sheet: First Aid for Choking (Conscious Infant)

Partner Check
Instructor Check

☐ ☐ **Determine if Infant Is Choking**

Determine if infant can cry, cough, or breathe.

Partner/Instructor says, "Infant cannot cry, cough, or breathe."

Rescuer shouts, "Help!"

☐ ☐ **Phone the EMS System for Help**

Tell someone to call for an ambulance.

Rescuer says, "Infant choking,
call _____."
(Local emergency number or Operator)

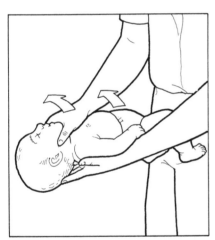

☐ ☐ **Give 4 Back Blows**

Grasp infant's jaw with your thumb and fingers.

Slide your other hand behind the infant's back so that your fingers support the back of the infant's head and neck.

Turn infant over so that infant is facedown on your forearm.

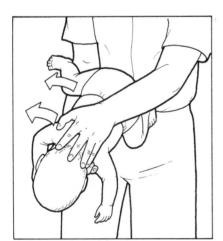

Support infant's head and neck with your hand by firmly holding the jaw between your thumb and fingers.

Lower your forearm onto your thigh. Infant's head should be lower than the chest.

Give 4 back blows forcefully between infant's shoulder blades with heel of your other hand.

Try to dislodge the object with each blow.

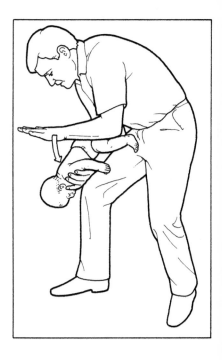

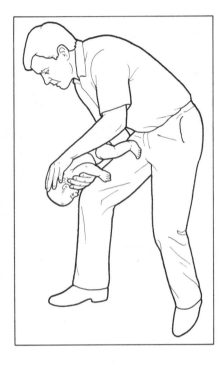

☐ ☐ **Give 4 Chest Thrusts**

Turn infant onto back.

Place your free hand and forearm along infant's head and back so that infant is sandwiched between your two hands and forearms.

Support back of infant's head and neck with your fingers.

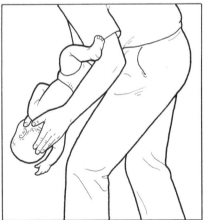

Turn infant onto his or her back, keeping head and body straight.

Lower your forearm onto your thigh.

Keep infant's head lower than his or her chest.

Locate position for chest thrusts.

Imagine a line running across infant's chest connecting nipples.

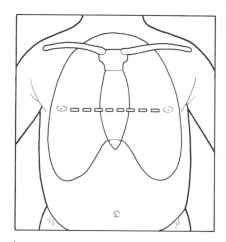

Place pad of ring finger on breastbone just below this imaginary line.

Place pads of next two fingers on breastbone beside the ring finger.

Pads of fingers should lie along length of breastbone.

Raise ring finger.

If you feel the notch at the end of the breastbone, move your fingers slightly toward the head.

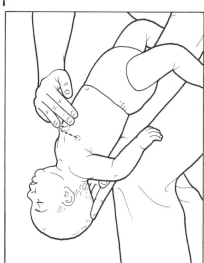

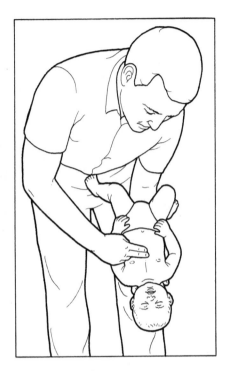

Partner Check   Instructor Check

Give 4 chest thrusts.

Using pads of two fingers, compress breastbone ½ to 1 inch (1.3 to 2.5 centimeters), 4 times.

Compress down and let up smoothly, keeping your fingers on the chest.

Try to dislodge the object with each thrust.

☐ ☐ **Repeat Back Blows and Chest Thrusts**

Continue giving back blows and chest thrusts until airway is clear or infant becomes unconscious.

Final Instructor Check_____

Skill Sheet: First Aid for Choking (Unconscious Infant)

You find an infant lying unusually still, and you suspect that something may be wrong. You should survey the scene to see if it is safe and to get some idea of what happened. Then do a primary survey.

Remember: **Do not do finger sweeps on a manikin. Do not touch a manikin's lips or inside the mouth with your fingers.**

Partner Check
Instructor Check

☐ ☐ **Check for Unresponsiveness** (Does the infant respond?)

Tap or gently shake infant's shoulder.

Partner/Instructor says, "Unconscious."

Rescuer repeats, "Unconscious."

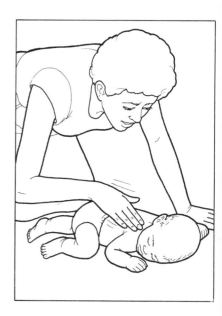

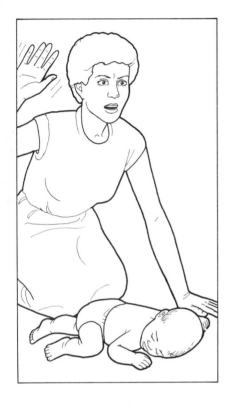

Partner Check
Instructor Check

Rescuer shouts, "Help!"

Position the Infant

Place the infant on his or her back.

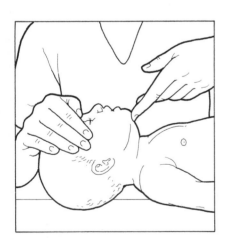

☐ ☐ **Open the Airway** (Use head-tilt/chin-lift.)

Put your hand—the one nearer the infant's head—on infant's forehead.

Put finger of other hand under bony part of lower jaw at the chin.

Tilt head gently back into the neutral position and lift chin.
Do not close infant's mouth completely. Do not push on the soft parts under the chin.

Partner Check
Instructor Check

☐ ☐ **Check for Breathlessness** (Is the infant breathing?)

Keep airway open with head-tilt/chin-lift.

Place your ear over infant's mouth and nose.

Look at chest and abdomen. Listen and feel for breathing for 3 to 5 seconds.

Partner/Instructor says, "No breathing."

Rescuer repeats, "No breathing."

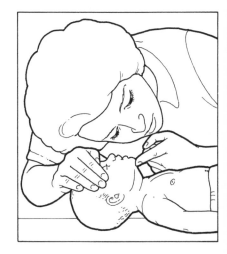

☐ ☐ **Give 2 Slow Breaths**

Keep airway open with head-tilt/chin-lift.

Open your mouth wide and take a breath. Seal your lips tightly around infant's mouth and nose.

Give 2 slow breaths. Each breath should last 1 to 1½ seconds. Take a breath yourself between the breaths you give the infant.

Partner/Instructor says, "Unable to breathe air into infant."

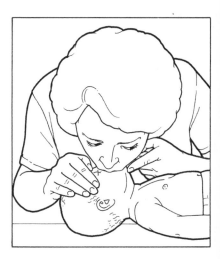

☐ ☐ **Retilt Infant's Head and Give 2 Slow Breaths**

Retilt infant's head and lift chin. Do not close infant's mouth completely. Do not push on the soft parts under the chin.

Open your mouth wide and take a breath. Seal your lips tightly around infant's mouth and nose.

Give 2 slow breaths. Each breath should last 1 to 1½ seconds. Take a breath yourself between the breaths you give the infant.

Partner/Instructor says, "Still unable to breathe air into infant."

Rescuer says, "Airway blocked."

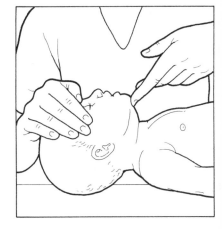

Partner Check
Instructor Check

☐ ☐ **Phone the EMS System for Help**

Tell someone to call for an ambulance.

Rescuer says, "Infant's airway blocked, call _____."
(Local emergency number or Operator)

☐ ☐ **Give 4 Back Blows**

Grasp infant's jaw with your thumb and fingers.

Slide your other hand behind the infant's back so that your fingers support the back of the infant's head and neck.

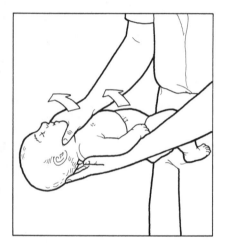

Turn infant over so that infant is facedown on your forearm.

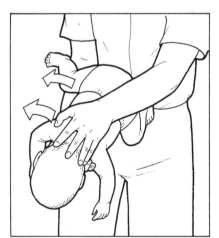

Partner Check
Instructor Check

Support infant's head and neck with your hand by firmly holding the jaw between your thumb and fingers.

Lower your forearm onto your thigh. Infant's head should be lower than the chest.

Give 4 back blows forcefully between infant's shoulder blades with heel of your other hand.

Try to dislodge the object with each blow.

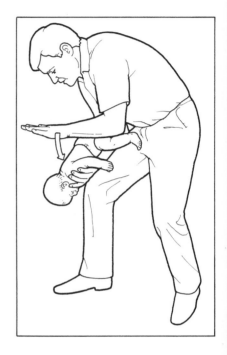

☐ ☐ **Give 4 Chest Thrusts**

Turn infant onto back.

Place your free hand and forearm along infant's head and back so that infant is sandwiched between your two hands and forearms.

Support back of infant's head and neck with your fingers.

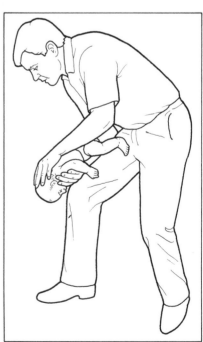

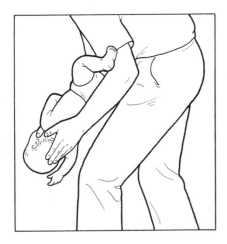

Turn infant onto his or her back, keeping head and body straight.

Lower your forearm onto your thigh.

Keep infant's head lower than his or her chest.

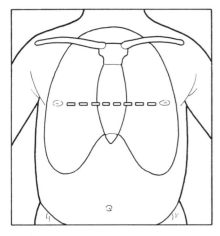

Locate position for chest thrusts.

Imagine a line running across infant's chest connecting nipples.

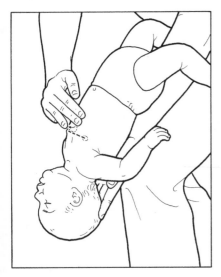

Place pad of ring finger on breastbone just below this imaginary line.

Place pads of next two fingers on breastbone beside the ring finger.

Pads of fingers should lie along length of breastbone.

Raise ring finger.

If you feel the notch at the end of the breastbone, move your fingers slightly toward the head.

Partner Check
Instructor Check

Give 4 chest thrusts.

Using pads of two fingers, compress breastbone ½ to 1 inch (1.3 to 2.5 centimeters), 4 times.

Compress down and let up smoothly, keeping your fingers on the chest.

Try to dislodge the object with each thrust.

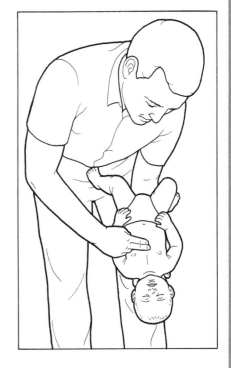

☐ ☐ **Foreign-Body Check** (Can you see an object in the throat?)

With infant's face up, open his or her mouth by grasping both tongue and lower jaw between thumb and fingers of hand nearer infant's legs. Lift jaw.

Look inside mouth for object. If you can see an object, try to remove it with a finger sweep.

Partner/Instructor says, "No object seen."

Rescuer repeats, "No object seen."

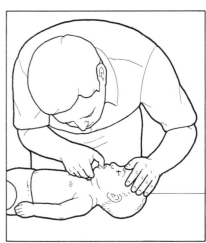

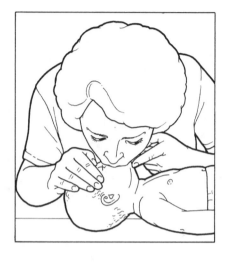

Partner Check
Instructor Check

☐ ☐ **Give 2 Slow Breaths**

Keep airway open with head-tilt/chin-lift.

Open your mouth wide and take a breath. Seal your lips tightly around infant's mouth and nose.

Give 2 slow breaths. Each breath should last 1 to 1½ seconds. Take a breath yourself between the breaths you give the infant.

Partner/Instructor says, "Airway still blocked."

☐ ☐ **Repeat Sequence**

Give 4 back blows.

Give 4 chest thrusts.

Do foreign-body check.

Give 2 slow breaths.

☐ ☐ **What to Do Next**

While the rescuer is repeating the sequence of back blows, chest thrusts, foreign-body check, and rescue breaths, the partner should read one of the following statements:

1. Rescuer can breathe into infant's lungs after doing foreign-body check.

2. After foreign-body check, object is removed with finger sweep.

3. Object is expelled during chest thrusts.

The rescuer should use this information to decide what to do next and then give the right care.

Final Instructor Check_____

Review Section: First Aid for Choking (Conscious Infant)

You are feeding your 10-month-old nephew. A loud noise scares him just as he has taken a spoonful of food, and he chokes. He cannot cry, cough, or breathe. You shout for help and have someone phone the EMS system.

1. What type of first aid should you give?
   - ☐ a. Chest compressions followed by rescue breaths
   - ☐ b. Back blows followed by chest thrusts
   - ☐ c. Abdominal thrusts followed by a foreign-body check

2. The infant coughs up the food.
   You should watch him carefully until _____ personnel arrive.

Answers

1. **b.** If a conscious infant has choked and cannot cry, cough, or breathe, you should give **back blows followed by chest thrusts.**

2. When the infant coughs up the food, you should watch him carefully until **EMS** personnel arrive.

Review Section: First Aid for Choking (Unconscious Infant)

You are watching TV and eating popcorn with a 10-year-old. His 8-month-old brother is crawling near you. You leave the room to answer the phone, and the boy comes running to tell you that there is something wrong with the infant. You find the infant lying on the floor, not moving. You check for unresponsiveness. He is unconscious. You position him on his back.

1. What should you do next?
   - ☐ a. Open the airway and check for breathing.
   - ☐ b. Give 4 back blows and 4 chest thrusts.
   - ☐ c. Give 1 rescue breath every 3 seconds.

You cannot breathe air into the infant when you give 2 slow breaths.

2. What should you do now?
   - ☐ a. Do a foreign-body check.
   - ☐ b. Give 6 to 10 abdominal thrusts.
   - ☐ c. Retilt the head and give 2 more slow breaths.

You still can't breathe air into the infant.

3. What should you do?
   - ☐ a. Give 4 back blows followed by 4 chest thrusts.
   - ☐ b. Give 6 to 10 abdominal thrusts.
   - ☐ c. Do a foreign-body check.

When doing a foreign-body check, you see an object in the infant's throat and remove it with a finger sweep.

4. What should you do next?
   - ☐ a. Check for a pulse.
   - ☐ b. Give 2 slow breaths.
   - ☐ c. Continue back blows and chest thrusts.

Answers

1. a. If the infant is unconscious, you should **open the airway and check for breathing.**

2. c. You should **retilt the head and give 2 more slow breaths** if you can't breathe air into the infant.

3. a. If you still can't breathe air into the infant, you should **give 4 back blows followed by 4 chest thrusts.**

4. b. After the object is removed, you should **give 2 slow breaths.**

8 *What to Do When an Infant's Heart Stops (CPR)*

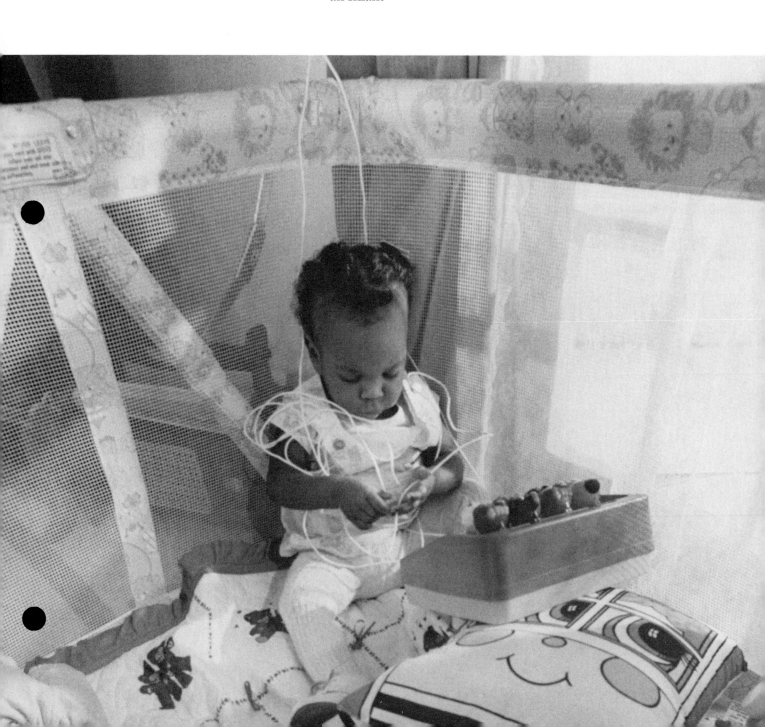

In Chapter 5, you learned how to give CPR to a child. In this chapter, you will learn how to give CPR to an infant younger than one year old. You will learn how to keep oxygen-carrying blood flowing through the infant's body.

Objectives

By the time you finish reading this chapter, you should be able to do the following:

1. *Describe when an infant needs CPR.*
2. *Explain why you must check the infant's brachial pulse before you start CPR.*
3. *Describe how to give CPR to an infant.*
4. *Explain when you should check to find out if the infant's heart is beating again after you start CPR.*
5. *List four conditions when a rescuer may stop CPR.*

Cardiac Emergencies in Infants

When an infant's heart stops beating, this is a cardiac emergency. The most common cause of cardiac emergencies in infants is sudden infant death syndrome (SIDS). SIDS is a sudden event. You cannot predict or prevent it.

Researchers have learned some things about SIDS—

- Ninety percent of SIDS deaths occur while the infant is asleep (between midnight and 8 a.m.).
- SIDS deaths can occur between the ages of two weeks and 18 months. The majority of deaths occur between one and six months of age.
- The majority of SIDS deaths occur in fall and winter.
- Thirty to 50 percent of SIDS victims have minor respiratory infections at the time of death.
- SIDS occurs slightly more often in boys than girls.

There are other causes of cardiac emergencies in infants besides SIDS. A cardiac emergency can happen when an infant is injured in a motor vehicle accident or suffers burns or electric shock. Poisoning, suffocation, and near-drowning can cause an infant's heart to stop. A cardiac emergency can happen when an infant's airway becomes blocked. Sometimes a medical condition or an illness, such as severe croup, leads to a cardiac emergency.

Except for SIDS, many cardiac emergencies in infants can be prevented since they are caused by injuries. Protecting infants from injury will prevent cardiac emergencies. Chapter 1 describes many ways you can reduce the risk of injury—for example, by always buckling an infant into an approved car safety seat. A second way to prevent cardiac emergencies is to make sure infants have the medical care they need.

A third way to prevent cardiac emergencies is to give first aid when an infant has a breathing emergency. The following signals are warnings that a breathing emergency may be about to happen:

- Infant is agitated.
- Infant is drowsy.
- Infant's skin color changes (to pale, blue, or gray).
- Infant is having difficulty breathing.
- Infant is breathing faster.
- Infant's heart is beating faster.

Unless a breathing emergency is recognized and treated, a cardiac emergency may develop. In this chapter, you will learn how to help an infant whose heart has stopped beating. When an infant's heart stops, you must give first aid right away. You must begin CPR to keep oxygen-carrying blood circulating through the body.

How to Give CPR to an Infant

Decide if the Infant Needs CPR

To find out if an infant needs CPR, start with a primary survey.
You should—

1. Check for unresponsiveness.
2. Shout for help.
3. Position the infant on his or her back.
4. Open the airway.
5. Look, listen, and feel for breathing for 3 to 5 seconds.
6. If the infant is not breathing, give 2 slow breaths.
7. Check the brachial pulse for heartbeat for 5 to 10 seconds.
8. Have someone phone the EMS system for help.

If the infant has no pulse, begin CPR. **It is important to check the infant's brachial pulse for 5 to 10 seconds before you start CPR. It is dangerous to do chest compressions if the infant's heart is beating.**

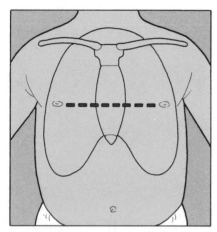

Figure 58
Imaginary Line Between Nipples

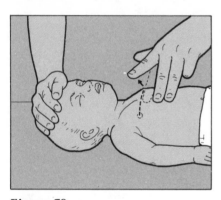

Figure 59
Position for Giving
Compressions

Position Yourself and the Infant

Both you and the infant must be in the correct position for CPR to work.

To position the infant—
- Lay the infant on his or her back on a firm, flat surface. The infant's head must be on the same level as the heart.

To position yourself—
- Stand or kneel facing the infant from the side.
- Use your hand—the one nearer the infant's head—to hold the head in the neutral position.
- Now find the compression point with your other hand. Imagine a line running across the chest between the infant's nipples *(Fig.58)*. Put the pad of your index finger on the breastbone just below this imaginary line.
- Put the pads of two fingers next to your index finger on the breastbone.
- Raise your index finger *(Fig. 59)*. If your fingers are in the correct position, you are less likely to break the infant's ribs.

Review Questions

Check the best answer(s).

1. When should you give CPR to an infant?
   - ☐ a. When an infant is not breathing and has no pulse
   - ☐ b. When an infant is not breathing but has a pulse
   - ☐ c. When an infant is choking

2. When you give CPR, an infant should be lying on a firm, flat surface. Which of the following would be suitable? (Check two.)
   - ☐ a. Crib
   - ☐ b. Couch
   - ☐ c. Floor
   - ☐ d. Table

Answers

1. **a.** You should give CPR **when an infant is not breathing and has no pulse.**

2. When you give CPR to an infant, the infant should be lying on a firm, flat surface such as—
   c. The **floor.**
   d. A **table.**

Give Chest Compressions

1. Use only the two fingers that are on the infant's breastbone **(Fig. 60).** Push straight down when you compress. Your elbow should be bent.

2. Each time you compress, push the infant's breastbone down from ½ to 1 inch (1.3 to 2.5 centimeters) **(Fig. 61).** Then release pressure.

3. Give smooth compressions. Keep a steady down-and-up pace. Do not pause between compressions. When you come up, release pressure on the infant's chest but keep your fingers on the breastbone.

4. Give compressions at the rate of at least 100 compressions per minute.

5. Do cycles of 5 compressions and 1 breath. Count out loud very quickly, "One, two, three, four, five." This will help you give compressions at the right rate. When you finish 5 compressions, keep your fingers in position on the infant's chest. Keep your other hand on the forehead. Give 1 slow breath.

6. If the infant's chest does not rise when you breathe in, you need to open the airway. Remove your fingers from the breastbone and lift the chin. Give 1 slow breath. Then put your fingers back on the breastbone in the compression position to continue cycles of 5 compressions and 1 breath.

7. After 10 cycles of 5 compressions and 1 breath, recheck the pulse. Remove your fingers from the chest and check the brachial pulse for 5 seconds. If there is no pulse, continue cycles of compressions and breaths.

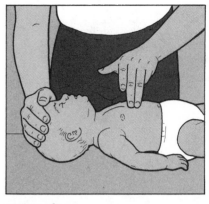

Figure 60
Give Chest Compressions

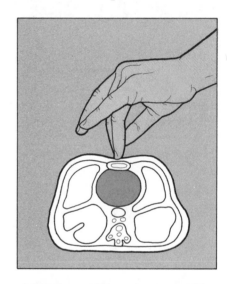

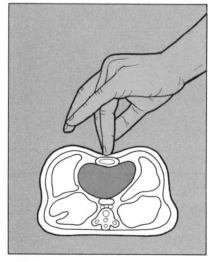

Figure 61
Compress Chest ½ to 1 inch

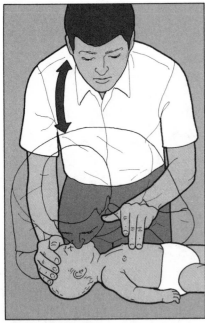

Figure 62
5 Compressions, Then 1 Breath

Put the Steps Together

Here are the steps for giving CPR to an infant:

1. Check for unresponsiveness.
2. Shout for help.
3. Position the infant on his or her back on a firm, flat surface.
4. Open the airway.
5. Look, listen, and feel for breathing for 3 to 5 seconds.
6. If the infant is not breathing, give 2 slow breaths.
7. Check the infant's brachial pulse for heartbeat for 5 to 10 seconds.
8. Tell someone to phone the EMS system for help.
9. If there is no pulse, find the correct finger position to give chest compressions.
10. Give 5 compressions without stopping, at the rate of at least 100 compressions per minute. Keep the infant's head in the neutral position with your other hand.
11. Give 1 slow breath. The breath should last 1 to 1½ seconds.
12. Keep repeating cycles of 5 compressions and 1 breath *(Fig. 62)*.
13. After 10 cycles of 5 compressions and 1 breath (about 1 minute), recheck the brachial pulse for 5 seconds.
14. If there is no pulse, give 1 breath and continue CPR. Recheck the pulse every few minutes.

    If there is a pulse, check for breathing for 3 to 5 seconds. If the infant is breathing, keep the airway open. Keep checking breathing and pulse closely. Look, listen, and feel for breathing. Check the pulse once every minute. Cover the infant. Keep the infant warm and as quiet as possible. If the infant is not breathing, give rescue breathing and keep checking the pulse once every minute.
15. Continue CPR until one of the following things happens:
    - The heart starts beating again.
    - A second rescuer trained in CPR takes over for you.
    - EMS personnel arrive and take over.
    - You are too exhausted to continue.

Review Questions

Check the best answer.

3. How far should you compress the chest of an infant?
- ☐ a. ½ to 1 inch (1.3 to 2.5 centimeters)
- ☐ b. 1 to 1½ inches (2.5 to 3.8 centimeters)
- ☐ c. 1½ to 2 inches (3.8 to 5 centimeters)

4. When you give CPR to an infant, at what rate should you give chest compressions?
- ☐ a. 50 to 60 times per minute
- ☐ b. 60 to 80 times per minute
- ☐ c. At least 100 times per minute

5. When you give CPR to an infant, what is the correct cycle?
- ☐ a. 5 compressions, then 1 breath
- ☐ b. 10 compressions, then 2 breaths
- ☐ c. 15 compressions, then 2 breaths

6. After starting CPR on an infant, when should you check for the return of pulse?
- ☐ a. Only after 4 cycles of CPR
- ☐ b. After 10 cycles of CPR and every few minutes thereafter
- ☐ c. After 15 cycles of CPR and every minute thereafter

Answers

3. a. You should compress the chest of an infant ½ **to 1 inch (1.3 to 2.5 centimeters).**

4. c. When you give CPR to an infant, you should give chest compressions at the rate of **at least 100 times per minute.**

5. a. When you give CPR to an infant, you should do cycles of **5 compressions, then 1 breath.**

6. b. After starting CPR on an infant, you should check for the return of pulse **after 10 cycles of CPR and every few minutes thereafter.**

More About CPR for an Infant

If No One Comes When You Shout for Help

When you find an unresponsive infant, always shout for help. Shout to attract someone nearby who can phone the EMS system for help. But what if no one comes when you shout for help? You should do CPR for at least one minute. Keep shouting for help. Also plan how to make the call yourself.

If no one comes to help you after one minute of CPR, you should go to a phone as quickly as you can and call the EMS system. If possible, bring the phone where the infant is or carry the infant with you to the phone. Begin CPR again after you have made the call.

If a Second Trained Rescuer Is at the Scene

If another person trained in CPR is at the scene, this person should do two things: first, phone the EMS system for help if this has not been done; and second, take over CPR when you are tired. The second person should say that he or she is trained in CPR and offer to help you. If the EMS system has been called and if you are tired and ask for help, then—

1. You should stop CPR after the next breath.
2. The second rescuer should stand or kneel beside the infant across from you. Then he or she should tilt the infant's head into the neutral position and feel for the brachial pulse for 5 seconds.
3. If there is no pulse, the second rescuer should give 1 breath and continue CPR.
4. You should check to make sure the second rescuer is doing CPR correctly. Watch the infant's chest rise and fall during rescue breathing, and feel for the brachial pulse. If you feel a pulse while compressions are being done, you know the compressions are being done correctly.

Practice Session: CPR for an Infant

During this practice session, you and a partner will practice on a manikin. **Before you start practicing,** carefully read the skill sheet on pages 176 through 182. If you don't remember how to use the skill sheet, read "Practice Sessions: Information and Directions" on pages 55 through 57.

Before you practice on the manikin, clean its face and the inside of its mouth. Directions for doing this are given in the section called "Some Health Precautions and Guidelines to Follow During This Course" on pages 3 and 4 of this workbook. **Clean the manikin's face and mouth before each person in your group practices.**

Skill Sheet: CPR for an Infant

You find an infant lying unusually still, and you suspect that something may be wrong. You should survey the scene to see if it is safe and to get some idea of what happened. Then do a primary survey.

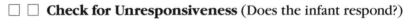

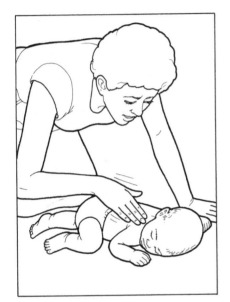

☐ ☐ **Check for Unresponsiveness** (Does the infant respond?)

Tap or gently shake infant's shoulder.

Partner/Instructor says, "Unconscious."

Rescuer repeats, "Unconscious."

Rescuer shouts, "Help."

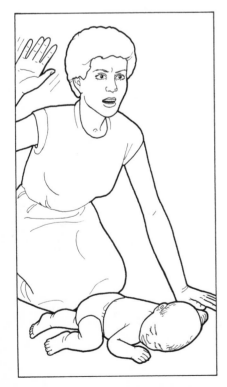

Position the Infant

Place the infant on his or her back.

Partner Check
Instructor Check

☐ ☐ **Open the Airway** (Use head-tilt/chin-lift.)

Put your hand—the one nearer the infant's head—on infant's forehead.

Put finger of other hand under bony part of lower jaw at the chin.

Tilt head gently back into neutral position and lift chin. Do not close the infant's mouth completely. Do not push on the soft parts under the chin.

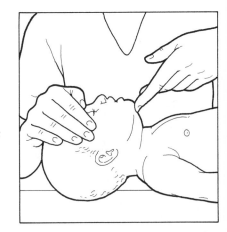

☐ ☐ **Check for Breathlessness** (Is the infant breathing?)

Keep airway open with head-tilt/chin-lift.

Place your ear over infant's mouth and nose.

Look at chest and abdomen. Listen and feel for breathing for 3 to 5 seconds.

Partner/Instructor says, "No breathing."

Rescuer repeats, "No breathing."

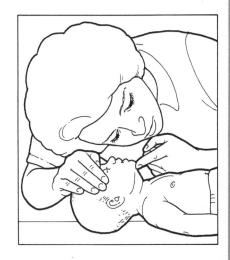

☐ ☐ **Give 2 Slow Breaths**

Keep airway open with head-tilt/chin-lift.

Open your mouth wide and take a breath. Seal your lips tightly around infant's mouth and nose.

Give 2 slow breaths. Each breath should last 1 to 1½ seconds. Take a breath yourself between the breaths you give the infant.

Look for the chest to rise and fall. Listen and feel for air coming out of infant's nose and mouth.

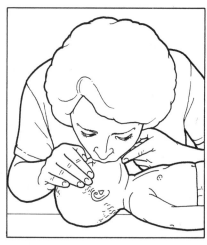

Partner Check
Instructor Check

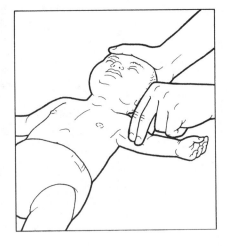

☐ ☐ **Check for Pulse**

Keep infant's head tilted with one hand on forehead.

With other hand press gently with your index and middle fingers on inside of upper arm.

Feel for brachial pulse for 5 to 10 seconds.

Partner/Instructor says, "No breathing and no pulse."

Rescuer repeats, "No breathing and no pulse."

☐ ☐ **Phone the EMS System for Help**

Tell someone to call for an ambulance.

Rescuer says, "Infant not breathing, has no pulse, call _____."
(Local emergency number or Operator)

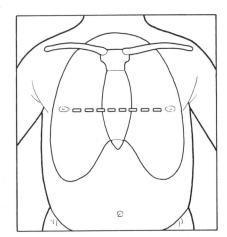

☐ ☐ **Find Compression Position**

Stand or kneel facing infant.

Keep infant's head tilted with hand on forehead.

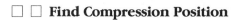

Imagine a line running across the chest connecting the nipples.

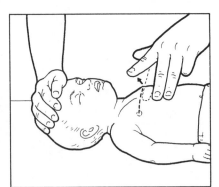

Place pad of your index finger on breastbone just below this imaginary line.

Place pads of two fingers next to your index finger on breastbone.

Pads of fingers should lie along the length of breastbone.

Raise your index finger.

If you feel the notch at the end of breastbone, move your fingers slightly toward the head.

Partner Check
Instructor Check

☐ ☐ **Give 5 Compressions**

Compress breastbone ½ to 1 inch (1.3 to 2.5 centimeters) at the rate of at least 100 compressions per minute (5 compressions should take 3 seconds or less).

Count out loud very quickly, "One, two, three, four, five."

Compress down and let up smoothly, keeping your fingers on the chest at all times.

Keep infant's head tilted with hand on forehead.

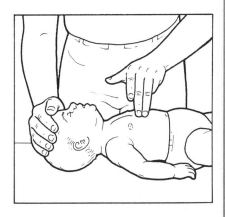

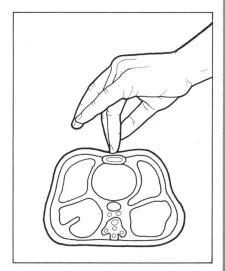

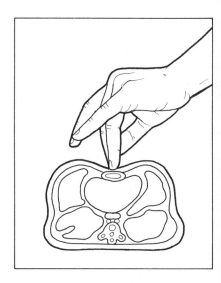

Partner Check
Instructor Check

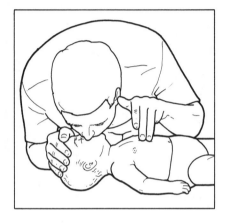

☐ ☐ **Give 1 Slow Breath**

Stop compressions. Keep fingers in position.

Keep infant's head tilted with hand on forehead.

Open your mouth wide and take a breath. Seal your lips tightly around infant's mouth and nose.

Give 1 slow breath. The breath should last 1 to 1½ seconds.

Look for the chest to rise and fall. Listen and feel for air coming out of the infant's mouth and nose.

If chest does not rise, use the hand on the infant's chest to lift the infant's chin and open the airway.

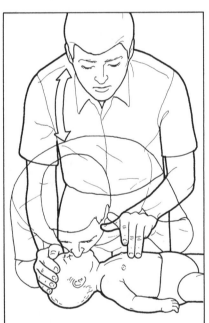

☐ ☐ **Do Compression/Breathing Cycles**

Keep infant's head tilted with one hand on forehead.

Do 10 cycles of 5 compressions and 1 breath.

Recheck pulse every few minutes.

180

Partner Check
Instructor Check

☐ ☐ **Recheck Pulse**

Keep infant's head tilted with one hand on forehead.

With other hand feel for brachial pulse for 5 seconds.

Partner/Instructor says, "No pulse."

Rescuer repeats, "No pulse."

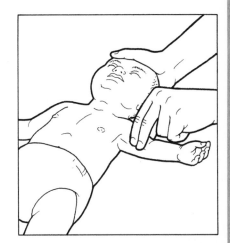

☐ ☐ **Give 1 Slow Breath**

Return hand to infant's chest. Locate compression point.

Keep infant's head tilted with hand on forehead.

Open your mouth wide and take a breath. Seal your lips tightly around infant's mouth and nose.

Give 1 slow breath. The breath should last 1 to 1½ seconds.

Look for the chest to rise and fall. Listen and feel for air coming out of the infant's mouth and nose.

If chest does not rise, use the hand on the infant's chest to lift the infant's chin and open the airway.

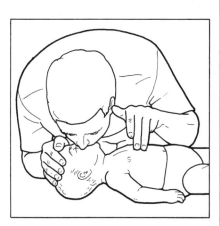

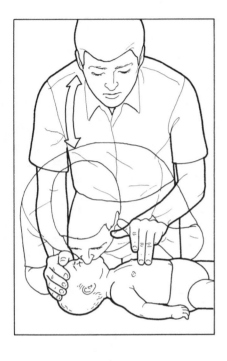

Partner Check
Instructor Check

☐ ☐ **Continue Compression/Breathing Cycles**

Continue cycles of 5 compressions and 1 breath.

Recheck pulse every few minutes.

☐ ☐ **What to Do Next**

When the rescuer stops to check pulse, the partner should read one of the following statements:

1. Infant has a pulse.

2. Infant does not have a pulse.

The rescuer should use this information to decide what to do next and then give the right care.

Final Instructor Check_____

Review Section: CPR for an Infant

You are at a family reunion. A boy runs into the house and says that his baby sister has fallen into the swimming pool. You rush into the yard and take the infant out of the pool. You check for unresponsiveness. She is unconscious.

1. What should you do now?
   - [ ] a. Check the ABCs.
   - [ ] b. Give back blows and chest thrusts.
   - [ ] c. Begin CPR.

You find that the infant is not breathing. You give 2 slow breaths. Then you check the brachial pulse in the upper arm. You do not feel a pulse. You begin CPR.

2. When giving CPR to an infant, at what rate should you compress the chest?
   - [ ] a. 50 to 60 times per minute
   - [ ] b. 70 to 80 times per minute
   - [ ] c. At least 100 times per minute

3. How far should you compress an infant's chest when giving CPR?
   - [ ] a. ½ to 1 inch (1.3 to 2.5 centimeters)
   - [ ] b. 1 to 1½ inches (2.5 to 3.8 centimeters)
   - [ ] c. 1½ to 2 inches (3.8 to 5 centimeters)

After doing 10 cycles (about 1 minute) of CPR, you recheck the infant's pulse for 5 seconds. There is no pulse.

4. What should you do?
   - [ ] a. Give 1 rescue breath every 4 seconds.
   - [ ] b. Continue CPR.
   - [ ] c. Keep the infant warm.

Answers

1. **a.** You should **check the ABCs** if the infant is unconscious.

2. **c.** When giving CPR to an infant, you should compress the chest at the rate of **at least 100 times per minute.**

3. **a.** When giving CPR to an infant, you should compress the infant's chest ½ **to 1 inch (1.3 to 2.5 centimeters).**

4. **b.** If there is no pulse when you recheck for pulse, you should **continue CPR.**

Appendixes

185

Throughout this course, you have learned how important it is for you and your community's EMS system to work together to give the victim of a medical emergency the best chance of survival.

This appendix explains what an EMS system is and how a victim of injury or sudden illness "enters" the system. It also explains the different types of care that a victim may require (basic life support and advanced life support) and what should happen when EMS personnel arrive at the scene of an emergency. At the end of this appendix there is a list of questions to help you learn more about your community's EMS system.

Objectives

By the time you finish reading this appendix, you should be able to do the following:

1. Describe the purpose of an Emergency Medical Services (EMS) system.

2. List at least three parts of an EMS system.

3. Describe the three main responsibilities of a trained citizen-rescuer when a medical emergency occurs.

4. List five facts that you should know about your community's EMS system.

What Is an Emergency Medical Services (EMS) System?

To save a life in a life-threatening situation, two things must happen. Emergency care must be started right away by a trained bystander, and this care must be continued and enhanced by EMS personnel when they arrive. If no one with first aid training is nearby to begin emergency care immediately, or if the community's EMS system cannot quickly provide the right kind of help, then a victim's chances of survival may be greatly reduced.

By taking this course, you have already taken one step to improve the ability of your community's EMS system to save lives. You have increased the chances that a trained person—you—may be able to help at the scene of an accident or other medical emergency until EMS personnel arrive. Your ability to provide care immediately could save a life.

Components of an EMS System

Providing the victim with the right care at the right time is not an easy task. Although most communities have some way of sending medical help to victims of sudden illness or accidents, this help may not include everything that the victim needs and may not arrive in time to give the victim the best chance of surviving. Your community's ability to get the right help to the victim as quickly as possible requires both planning and resources. Effective EMS systems usually have the following parts:

1. **Trained citizens.** Trained citizens like you can give first aid and alert the EMS system that a medical emergency has happened.

2. **Trained personnel.** To provide the best help quickly, an EMS system has specially trained personnel. These may include emergency medical technicians (EMTs), emergency medical technician-paramedics (paramedics), first responders (police, firefighters), emergency dispatchers, and hospital emergency department physicians and nurses trained in emergency medicine.

3. **Special equipment.** Specialized medical, rescue, and transportation equipment is required for various situations.

4. **Communications systems.** How well the EMS system works depends on how quickly citizens can alert the system that an emergency has happened and how quickly the EMS dispatcher can get the appropriate emergency personnel to the scene. Communications systems are also important because EMS personnel often need to communicate with the hospital emergency department as they care for the victim at the scene of the emergency and on the way to the hospital.

5. **Management and evaluation.** An EMS system needs a management structure that includes administration and coordination of all parts of the system, medical supervision and direction, and ongoing evaluation and research.

The Responsibilities of the Rescuer in the EMS System

In order for the victim of a medical emergency to receive care from the EMS system, the victim must **enter** the system. This means that the EMS system must be told about the emergency. Then, until EMS personnel arrive, the victim should receive the proper first aid. These important first steps are generally performed by a citizen-rescuer. There are three things that **you** must do to make sure that a victim enters the EMS system, with the best chance for survival:

1. **Recognize that a medical emergency has happened.** This isn't always easy. Medical problems are not always obvious, but the skills you have learned in this course will help you recognize emergencies.

2. **Give first aid (basic life support).** You have been trained to provide first aid for breathing and cardiac emergencies. CPR, rescue breathing, and first aid for choking are all basic life support techniques.

3. **Phone the EMS system for help.** You may phone or direct bystanders to phone for help. Give all necessary information so that appropriate medical care can reach the scene of the emergency. This information is discussed in Chapter 2.

How an EMS System Responds to a Call for Help

In many communities, a dispatcher will answer your call. The dispatcher is very important in making sure that the victim gets the right care immediately. In some systems, this person has special training to get specific information from the caller and to know which personnel and equipment to send to the scene. Some dispatchers can also give first aid instructions to the caller over the phone when it is necessary.

Basic Life Support and Advanced Life Support

As explained in Chapter 2, the information you provide to the EMS dispatcher is important. It will help determine the type of care that the dispatcher sends to the scene of an emergency. The dispatcher may send either an ambulance capable of continuing **basic life support** or an ambulance capable of delivering **advanced life support.** The care sent will depend on the needs of the victim and the services available in your community.

Most requests for emergency medical services require basic life support. For this reason, many states require that all ambulances be staffed with personnel trained to provide at least basic life support.

Some requests for assistance also require advanced life support. For example, a victim of a heart attack or cardiac arrest requires both basic life support and advanced life support. Advanced life support personnel may be supervised by a hospital-based physician.

A key thing to remember is that basic life support and advanced life support must be given within specific time periods to give the victim the best chance of survival. This is why it is important to have a well-coordinated EMS system in your community. Highly trained personnel can do more to help the victim if they arrive promptly.

First Responders

When a dispatcher receives a call for emergency medical help, he or she will select the type of care that is needed and send the appropriate personnel. This may include police, fire, rescue, and ambulance personnel, depending on the type of emergency and the resources available at the time of the call.

In many communities, police and firefighters may arrive at the scene before the ambulance because they are often located closer to the scene of the emergency. If you have been caring for a victim, the "first responder" may take over or ask you to assist. On the other hand, the first responder may tell you to continue care while he or she attends to other problems at the scene. It is important that you do not stop caring for a victim until the first responder takes over. You should expect the first responder to ask you for information about the victim. Information that you have gained from the primary and secondary surveys of the victim may be valuable to first responders, EMTs, paramedics, and to the hospital staff who will care for the victim later.

When the Ambulance Arrives

When the ambulance arrives, the EMTs or paramedics will take over responsibility for care of the victim and will provide additional medical care. Their goal is to begin to stabilize the victim's condition (correct life-threatening problems) at the scene. Once this has been done, the EMS personnel will prepare the victim for transport to the appropriate hospital emergency department, and they will continue caring for the victim on the way. When the ambulance arrives at the hospital, the EMS personnel will transfer responsibility for care of the victim to the emergency department staff.

You and Your EMS System

As you can see, the process by which you and the EMS system work together to save a life is complex. You should know that many communities do not have EMS systems that contain all of the features described above.

If you have ever been concerned about someone close to you having a heart attack or being the victim of a medical emergency, you owe it to yourself to find out what type of care your community's EMS system can provide **before** an emergency happens. When minutes count, your knowledge of your community's EMS system can help you make the right decisions. The following checklist has been included to help you find out more about your community's EMS system.

A Guide to Assessing Your Community's Emergency Medical Services (EMS) System

The following questions reflect the EMS standards set forth in the Emergency Medical Services Systems Act of 1973, the federal EMS legislation.

1. Are regularly scheduled CPR and first aid classes, open to the public, offered in your community? Yes_____ No_____

2. Does your community have a 911 emergency number for EMS, fire, and police? Yes_____ No_____

3. Do your local schools certify students in first aid and CPR? Yes_____ No_____

4. Are local police officers trained and certified in American Red Cross First Aid or in the U.S. Department of Transportation First Responder training? Yes_____ No_____

5. Is your local ambulance service staffed by EMTs? Yes_____ No_____

6. Does your local ambulance service regularly leave the station to answer an emergency call within two minutes of receiving the call? Yes_____ No_____

7. Does your community have advanced life support units staffed by emergency medical technician-paramedics? Yes_____ No_____

8. Are rescue services in your community (EMS, police, fire) provided by well-equipped units staffed by EMTs? Yes_____ No_____

9. Are all emergency services in your community dispatched and coordinated through a central emergency communications center? Yes_____ No_____

10. Is your nearest hospital emergency department staffed on a 24-hour basis by physicians and nurses who are specially trained in emergency medicine? Yes_____ No_____

11. Does your community have a plan to transfer acutely ill or badly injured patients to specialty centers? Yes_____ No_____

12. Does your community have an area-wide disaster plan to deal with multi-casualty incidents, natural disasters, and environmental emergencies? Yes_____ No_____

13. Is there one office in charge of the administration, coordination, and evaluation of the EMS system? Yes_____ No_____

Adapted from *A Community Scoring Guide for Emergency Health Services*, Office of Emergency Medical Services, The Pennsylvania State University.

With a better idea of the different parts and responsibilities of a community emergency medical services system, you will be better able to assess the emergency medical services offered by your own community.

Your answers to the preceding questions will help you evaluate the services that your community provides. The questions to which you have answered "Yes" will show you the strengths of your community's EMS system. The questions to which you have answered "No" will point out areas where your community's EMS system could be strengthened. As a citizen and a taxpayer, your support of your community's EMS system is as important as your knowing how to perform first aid.

Home Safety Checklist

Use this checklist to spot dangers in your home. When you read each question, mark the "Yes" box if your answer is "yes." Mark the "No" box if your answer is "no." Each mark in a "No" box shows a possible danger for you and your family. Work with your family to remove dangers and make your home safer.

Yes　　**No**

Outside the home

☐　☐　Is trash kept in tightly covered containers?
☐　☐　Are walkways, stairs, and railings in good repair?
☐　☐　Are walkways and stairs free of toys, tools, etc.?
☐　☐　Are sandboxes, wading pools, etc. covered when not in use?

Kitchen

☐　☐　Are pot handles turned inward when cooking?
☐　☐　Are hot dishes kept away from edge of table or counter?
☐　☐　Are hot foods and liquids kept out of child's reach?
☐　☐　Are knives and other sharp items kept out of child's reach?
☐　☐　Is high chair placed away from stove or other hot appliances?
☐　☐　Are matches and lighters kept out of child's reach?
☐　☐　Are all appliance cords kept out of child's reach?
☐　☐　Are cabinets equipped with safety latches?
☐　☐　Are cabinet doors kept closed when not in use?
☐　☐　Are cleaning products kept out of child's reach?

Bathroom

☐　☐　Are the toilet seat and lid kept down when not in use?
☐　☐　Are cabinets equipped with safety latches?
☐　☐　Are cabinet doors closed when not in use?
☐　☐　Are all medicines in child-resistant containers?
☐　☐　Are all medicines stored in a locked medicine cabinet?
☐　☐　Are shampoos and cosmetics stored out of child's reach?
☐　☐　Are razors, razor blades, and other sharp objects kept out of child's reach?
☐　☐　Are hairdryers and other appliances stored away from sink, tub, and toilet?
☐　☐　Does the bottom of tub or shower have rubber stickers or a rubber mat to prevent slipping?

Appendix: Home Safety Checklist

Yes   **No**

Child's room

☐ ☐ Is child's bed or crib placed away from radiators or other heated surfaces?
☐ ☐ Are crib slats no more than 2⅜ inches apart?
☐ ☐ Does mattress fit sides of crib snugly?
☐ ☐ Is paint on furniture nontoxic?
☐ ☐ Are electric cords kept out of child's reach?
☐ ☐ Does toy box have a safety hinge or cover?
☐ ☐ Are toys in good repair?
☐ ☐ Do toys have nontoxic finishes?
☐ ☐ Are toys appropriate for the child's age?
☐ ☐ Is child's clothing, especially sleepwear, flame resistant?

Parent's bedroom

☐ ☐ Are space heaters kept away from curtains and flammable materials?
☐ ☐ Are cosmetics stored out of child's reach?

Storage areas

☐ ☐ Are pesticides, detergents, and other household chemicals kept out of child's reach?
☐ ☐ Are tools kept out of child's reach?

General precautions inside the home

☐ ☐ Are stairways kept clear and uncluttered?
☐ ☐ Are stairs and hallways well lit?
☐ ☐ Are safety gates installed at tops and bottoms of stairways?
☐ ☐ Are rugs and runners skidproof?
☐ ☐ Are guards installed around fireplaces, radiators or hot pipes, and wood-burning stoves?
☐ ☐ Are sharp edges of furniture cushioned with corner guards or other material?
☐ ☐ Are unused electric outlets covered with tape or safety covers?
☐ ☐ Are curtain cords and shade pulls kept out of child's reach?
☐ ☐ Are windows secured with window locks?
☐ ☐ Are plastic bags kept out of child's reach?
☐ ☐ Are fire extinguishers installed where they are most likely to be needed?
☐ ☐ Are smoke detectors in working order?
☐ ☐ Do you have an emergency exit plan to use in case fire?

Yes	No	
☐	☐	Does your family practice using this emergency exit plan?
☐	☐	Is thermostat on water heater set to 120°F?
☐	☐	If you have a firearm, is it locked up where your child cannot get it?
☐	☐	Are all handbags, including those of visitors, kept out of child's reach?
☐	☐	Are all poisonous plants kept out of child's reach?
☐	☐	Is a list of instructions and important emergency phone numbers posted near phone?
☐	☐	Is a list of instructions posted near phone for use by children who are home alone?
☐	☐	Do you have syrup of ipecac in your home for use as directed in poisoning emergencies?

Glossary

Abdominal thrust—an upward push to the abdomen given to clear the airway of a person with a blocked airway. Also called the Heimlich maneuver.

Adam's apple—the protruding part in the front of the neck formed by the thyroid cartilage. To find the carotid pulse, you must first find the Adam's apple.

Airway—the passageway through which air enters the body and goes to the lungs.

Arteries—the blood vessels that carry blood away from the heart to the cells of the body.

Back blow—blow delivered with the heel of your hand between the shoulder blades of an infant. It is used along with chest thrusts to give first aid to an infant who is choking.

Blood vessels—the tubes through which blood circulates throughout the body.

Brachial pulse—the beat that is felt on the inside of an infant's upper arm. It is checked to determine the presence or absence of heartbeat. See **pulse.**

Breastbone—the main bone in the front, center part of the chest to which the ribs are connected.

Breathing emergency—a condition in which normal breathing is difficult or absent.

Breathlessness—the absence of breathing.

CPR—the abbreviation for cardiopulmonary resuscitation.

Cardiac emergency—a life-threatening condition in which the heart stops beating or the heartbeat becomes abnormal.

Cardiopulmonary resuscitation (CPR)—an emergency procedure used for a person who is not breathing and whose heart has stopped beating. The procedure involves a combination of chest compressions and rescue breathing.

Carotid pulse—the beat that is felt at the side of the neck when the carotid artery is pressed. Located between the windpipe and the neck muscle, the carotid pulse is checked to determine the presence or absence of heartbeat. See **pulse.**

Chest compression—a procedure for manually circulating blood in a person whose heart has stopped beating. It involves pressing down and letting up on the lower half of the breastbone. CPR is the combination of chest compressions and rescue breathing.

Chest thrust—a thrust to the middle of the breastbone that is used to clear the airway. Chest thrusts are used to give first aid to an infant who is choking.

Child—a person one through eight years old (for the purposes of this course).

Circulatory system—the system that carries blood to all parts of the body. The main parts of the circulatory system are the blood vessels and the heart.

Croup—a condition of the larynx. A child with croup has difficult and noisy breathing and a hoarse cough.

Decontamination—a thorough cleansing to reduce germs and contaminants.

EMS—the abbreviation for emergency medical services.

EMS dispatcher—a member of the emergency medical services (EMS) system who receives emergency calls and directs the appropriate personnel and equipment to the scene of a medical emergency.

Emergency action principles (EAP)—the four basic steps to follow in all emergency situations to ensure that victims receive proper care.

Emergency medical services (EMS) system—a community-based system that delivers specialized care for victims who are ill or injured. Care is provided at the scene of the emergency and is continued during transportation and following arrival at an appropriately staffed and equipped health care facility.

Finger pad—the underside of the fingertip. The pads of two fingers are used to compress the breastbone of a choking infant or an infant needing CPR.

Finger sweep—a technique used as part of the procedure to dislodge and remove a piece of food or an object from the airway of an unconscious choking victim.

Foreign body—an object that lodges in a person's airway, blocking the airway.

Foreign-body check—a procedure to determine if an object is lodged in an unconscious child's or infant's airway. If the object is visible, an attempt is made to remove it using the finger sweep.

Head-tilt/chin-lift—a technique used to open the airway of an unconscious person. It is done by applying backward pressure on the forehead and lifting the jaw. This tilts the head back and lifts the chin.

Heimlich maneuver—see **abdominal thrust.**

Implied consent—a legal term used to describe the assumption that an unconscious person, if he or she were conscious, would give consent to a rescuer to provide first aid. When the victim is an unconscious or severely injured child or infant, it is assumed that the parent or guardian would consent to first aid.

Infant—a person between birth and one year old (for the purposes of this course).

Infectious disease—a disease that may be transmitted or spread; a contagious disease.

Injury-prevention plan—a plan to reduce the risk of injury to infants and children by removing dangers, giving supervision, and teaching safety.

Manikin—a life-size model of a person used for practicing first aid skills for breathing and cardiac emergencies.

Mouth-to-mouth breathing—a form of rescue breathing in which a rescuer breathes air into the mouth and lungs of a person who is not breathing.

Mouth-to-nose breathing—a form of rescue breathing in which a rescuer breathes air into the nose and lungs of a person who is not breathing. This is done when injuries or other difficulties make it impossible to perform mouth-to-mouth breathing.

Mouth-to-stoma breathing—a form of rescue breathing in which a rescuer breathes air into the stoma and lungs of a person who is not breathing.

Nausea—a feeling of sickness in the stomach with an urge to vomit.

Neutral-plus position—the range of positions in which a child's head may be placed to open the airway.

Neutral position—the position in which an infant's head is placed to open the airway.

Notch—the place where the lower ribs meet the lower end of the breastbone in the center of the chest. Used as a reference point for finding the correct hand position in CPR.

911—a special telephone number used in many communities to give fast, direct connection to police, fire, and emergency medical services.

Oxygen—a gas that the cells of the body need in order to live. The air we breathe contains about 21 percent oxygen.

Oxygen-carrying blood—blood that contains oxygen.

Primary survey—a series of checks to discover conditions that are an immediate threat to a victim's life.

Pulmonary—having to do with the lungs.

Pulse—the rhythmic "beat" in an artery. As the heart pumps blood, the walls of the arteries expand and contract, causing a beat or a pulse. This beat or pulse can be felt by pressing on an artery.

Rescue breathing—the process of breathing air into the lungs of a person who has stopped breathing. Also called artificial respiration.

Rescuer—a person trained to survey the scene of an emergency, determine the extent of injuries, and provide first aid until EMS personnel arrive.

Respiratory system—the body system that draws air into the body and expels waste gases. The main parts are the airway and the lungs.

Resuscitation—an effort to artificially restore or provide normal heart and/or lung function.

Secondary survey—a series of checks to discover conditions that are not an immediate threat to a victim's life, but that may become life threatening if not corrected. These checks are done after life-threatening injuries have been found and cared for.

SIDS—the abbreviation for sudden infant death syndrome.

Sudden infant death syndrome—death of an apparently healthy infant due to unknown causes. Also called crib death.

Stoma—a surgically created opening in the front of the neck through which a person breathes.

Unresponsiveness—a condition in which a person does not react to verbal or physical stimuli.

Index

Index

Instructions for Emergency Phone Calls

Emergency Telephone Numbers

EMS_____ Fire_____ Police_____

Poison Control Center_____

Other Important Telephone Numbers

Doctor's name and number_____

Mother's name_____ Work number_____

Father's name_____Work number _____

Neighbor's name_____Home number_____

Name and address of medical facility with 24-hour emergency

cardiac care_____

_____

*   *   *   *   *

Information for Emergency Call (Be prepared to give this information to the EMS dispatcher.)

1. Location

   Street address_____

   City or town_____

   Directions (cross streets, landmarks, etc.)_____

   _____

2. Telephone number from which the call is being made
3. Caller's name
4. What happened
5. How many persons injured
6. Condition of victim(s)
7. Help (first aid) being given

Note: Do not hang up first. Let the EMS dispatcher hang up first.